PREVENTION

PREVENTION
The Ultimate Cure

Bill Little

PELICAN PUBLISHING COMPANY
Gretna 2006

Copyright © 1995
By Bill L. Little
All rights reserved

First published as *Eight Ways to Take an Active Role in Your Health*
   by WaterBrook Press, a division of Random House, Inc., 1995
Published by arrangement with the author by
   Pelican Publishing Company, Inc., 2006

The word "Pelican" and the depiction of a pelican are trademarks of Pelican Publishing Company, Inc., and are registered in the U.S. Patent and Trademark Office.

Library of Congress Cataloging-in-Publication Data

Little, Bill, 1935-
   Prevention : the ultimate cure / Bill Little.
   ISBN-13: 978-1-58980-413-5
   1. Health. 2. Self-care, Health. 3. Health attitudes.
4. Mind and body. I. Title.
RA776.5.L56 1995
613—dc20   95-2546
                                                                                  CIP

All Scripture quotations, unless otherwise indicated, are from *The Holy Bible, New International Version*®. NIV® copyright © 1973, 1978, 1984 International Bible Society. Used by permission of Zondervan Publishing House. All rights reserved.

Scripture quotations marked NASB are from the *New American Standard Bible,* Copyright © 1960, 1962, 1963, 1968, 1971, 1972, 1973, 1975, 1977 by the Lockman Foundation. Used by permission.

Scripture quotations marked KJV are from the King James Version of the Bible.

Printed in the United States of America

Published by Pelican Publishing Company, Inc.
1000 Burmaster Street, Gretna, Louisiana 70053

To my grandchildren, Candace, Shaun, Tyler, Anthony, Christian, Andrew, and Jack, and my great-grandson, Conner

Acknowledgements

It will be impossible to acknowledge all who helped make this book possible. There will be omissions in this list, but they are entirely unintentional.

Thanks first to a man who has given encouragement, put up with my phone calls, and spent a great deal of time and effort helping me edit the original manuscript. He is Floyd Thatcher from Waco, Texas. I can honestly say that without his patient and kind help, this manuscript would never have reached the publishers. I thank Floyd from the bottom of my heart.

Thanks also to the cancer patients who have encouraged me in this writing. Some of them have given permission for their names to be used in this manuscript. There are honestly too many to list. I am grateful to them for trusting me to work with them.

I especially thank my good friend and coworker at The Cancer Support Center of St. Louis, Administrative Director Gay Calstrom. Her helpful suggestions are sprinkled throughout the pages of this book.

I thank others who helped with the manuscript and correspondence. This refers to secretaries, Debbie Sage and Jan Viau. Special thanks to Susan Miller and Sandra Ash for proofreading and for helpful suggestions.

Finally, thanks to the people of the Christ Memorial Baptist Church in St. Louis. They have patiently encouraged me in expressing my thoughts for more than thirty-six years.

Contents

Preface 8

1 Facts and Fantasies 11
2 A True Story Is the Best Story 18
3 Step One: Choose to Live 32
4 Step Two: Adopt Healthy Beliefs 40
5 Step Three: Find Meaning 60
6 Step Four: Control Stress 69
7 Step Five: Develop Good Nutrition ... 85
8 Step Six: Celebrate Life 93
9 Step Seven: Envision Wholeness 104
10 Step Eight: Exercise Healthy Spirituality 119
11 The Last Word 141

Appendix A: Daily Thoughts on the Eight Steps 146

Appendix B: Special Guide for Cancer Patients 207

Preface

I have worked with people in counseling and healthcare since the 1960s. During that time I have had a growing conviction that we fail miserably at preventing all kinds of problems, especially health problems. If indeed disease and health are affected more by lifestyle than any other factor or combination of factors, then we can become active participants in protecting our own health.

While thinking about these issues, I came across three books that confirmed my thoughts. Glenn Clark wrote, "The first requirement for health is to love the spirit of health, which is wholeness. . . . The way to have a healthy body is to love the body, but in a pure, holy, spiritual way. When you begin to see the whole body, and love it, you will be amazed, not only to see how every organ, every nerve, every artery has an integral part in the health of your whole system, but how the body of your thoughts and emotions—your fear and faith, your jealousy and joy, your prejudice and pride, your laughter and love—all manifest sooner or later in the health states of your body" (*I Will Lift Up Mine Eyes,* pp. 144-45).

This concept fit perfectly with the ideas presented by Lawrence LaShan in *You Can Fight for Your Life.* This is a book about emotional causation in cancer.

I was growing to believe that there was a definite link between lifestyle and sickness.

The third book that helped blaze the trail to prevention for me was Carl and Stephanie Simonton's landmark *Getting Well Again*. They wrote, "Everyone participates in his or her health or illness at all times.... We all participate in our own health through our beliefs, our feelings, and our attitudes toward life, as well as in more direct ways, such as through exercise and diet" (p. 1).

It was in *Getting Well Again* that I first read ideas concerning visualization, stress reduction, and participation in healing, ideas that I have since seen in books by Bernie Siegel and Harold Benjamin, among others.

After reading these materials, I decided to write a mission statement for my life. I wrote, "My mission is to find and alleviate human suffering whenever I can and to have as much fun in the process as possible."

That mission statement led to a research project with cancer patients and ultimately to the writing of this book.

The principles contained here are healthy. They help us to heal when we are ill and, even more to my purpose, they help us prevent disease. One challenge that confronts us in the field of prevention is personal motivation. Even if a desire to take care of your own health doesn't motivate you, perhaps the awareness of cost savings will. Prevention is the ultimate way to reduce the cost of healthcare. Prevention is the ultimate cure.

Chapter 1

Facts and Fantasies

This book is about taking a proactive approach to health care. Most of us don't do that. We tend to be passive people, accepting what medical authorities tell us without question. Why?

Old Ideas Die Hard

I think Norman Cousins hit on some of the reasons in his book, *Head First*. There he lists five basic misconceptions that have dominated and distorted much thinking about health. The truth is that much of what we accept as "fact" is really misconception, and when we change our thinking we find out that we have a more active role to play in our health. Let's look at today's view of these misconceptions.

Misconception #1: Almost all illnesses are caused by disease germs or other external factors. We now know that disease is more than a matter of germs and other external factors. Many people may be exposed to the same germs, but not all of them will become ill. Part of the reason for this is genetic: We inherit some of our resistance to disease. But the environment also plays a role, and so does lifestyle (stress levels, how we think, what we eat, how much we have exercised, how we picture ourselves, how much we enjoy life, our sense of purpose, and our faith).

Louis Pasteur said disease was the result of germs (microbes). Claude Bernard thought the body's own equilibrium and internal environment were more important than microbes. Pasteur had the "facts" of science as they were recognized in his day. Bernard had theories and guesses. Yet it is reported that, on his deathbed, Pasteur said, "Bernard was right. The microbe is nothing; the soil is everything." Today we accept Bernard's theory as fact—disease is not simply a matter of germs.

Misconception #2: Illness proceeds in a straight line unless interrupted by outside intervention in one form or another. Today we know this is false. Illness does not simply progress in a straight line. Literature is filled with stories of spontaneous remission of disease. Some people get well without benefit of intervention.

Misconception #3: Pain is always a manifestation of disease, and the elimination of pain is therefore a manifestation of a return of good health. Norman Cousins points out that while we "make the mistake of equating pain with disease, very little is said about the fact that most pain belongs to a warning system to tell us that we are doing something wrong." Pain is not always a sign of disease. Sometimes it is telling us to not eat so much, stop smoking, or stop drinking too much.

Misconception #4: What goes into the mind has little or no effect on the body (and vice versa). There is little question now that what goes into the mind has a tremendous effect on health. Bill Moyers' documentary "How the Mind Heals the Body" is testimony to the newsworthiness of the mind-body connection. Further, Lawrence LaShan demonstrated in *You Can Fight For Your Life* that emotions are involved even in the development of cancer. Yes, the mind and body are one.

Misconception #5: Old age is connected to numbers of years—it begins at sixty-five, mental and physical abilities beyond that point fall off significantly, and society is justified in mandating retirement on the basis of age. But all of us know older people who seem to have more health and vigor than we do! The aerobics pioneer, Kenneth Cooper, M.D., recently stated in a lecture at the Aerobics Center in Dallas, Texas, that "though we cannot control the fact that our bodies age, we can control the rate at which they age." Cousins affirms that "recognition is growing that rapid aging is a disease that can be brought under greater control."

Someone Who Took Control

Denying these misconceptions means affirming our right and responsibility to take an active role in our own health care. It means no longer acting as passive participants in health but taking control. A friend, Judy Hunt, did just that.

Some time ago Judy sensed she had a lump in her breast. Her gynecologist thought she was unduly concerned, but requested a mammogram. It was judged to be clear, and she was so informed.

Though Judy respected this opinion, she knew her own body and had a sense that there was an increase in the size of her left breast. She went to a medical oncologist who chided her for being alarmist. He suggested that she come back in a year for another mammogram.

She was persistent. She insisted on a second examination by her gynecologist. The second exam coincided with the tenth day of her menstrual cycle, the most reliable time for a breast exam. This time the physician found a "possible lump." He suggested waiting 6 months and doing another exam.

Again she insisted, and a needle aspiration was done to distinguish between a fluid-filled cyst and a solid tumor. She writes, "As the procedure progressed, I observed the changing expression on my doctor's face. He didn't have to tell me that there was no fluid. My worst fears were realized when, following the biopsy, the surgeon said the word, 'malignant.'"

The surgeon suggested a mastectomy within a week. Judy asked about alternatives and was told that she was not a candidate for lumpectomy. But Judy wasn't convinced. She read materials from a cancer information center and found that the prognosis for lumpectomy followed by radiation was the same as for mastectomy. She opted for a lumpectomy, removal of tissue around the tumor and underarm lymph nodes, and radiation. She has a ninety-five percent likelihood of no recurrence.

Judy says, "I still have my own two breasts, with only one small scar to show that the left one was once cancerous. I don't want to discredit any physician, but I wish to encourage the reader to accept the ultimate responsibility for your own health. You are the one most qualified to make decisions relating to your body. To make such decisions, you must learn about the options available to you." If Judy had listened to the first two opinions, she might now be dealing with tumors that had spread beyond the breast. Judy took an active role in her own health care, and the outcome was much more satisfying to her as a result.

Get the Facts

This story illustrates several of the major points of this book. In making decisions about our health we must first ask questions. We have the right to ask our physicians for information. Ask, and if at first we don't get an answer, we must ask again! To get good information, we must get over our reluctance to ask physicians specific questions. Of course, we also have the right not to ask, but it should be a conscious choice, not the result of being afraid to ask.

Besides consulting a physician we can also ask other people who have been through what we're facing. What do they know? What advice do they have? And what advice do healthy friends have? What do they think keeps them healthy?

Judy got a second opinion, and a third one! She wasn't satisfied with just one person's view when it differed from her own. She was persistent until she found a doctor who was willing to do as she asked. Physicians are human beings, and most of them have no desire to be cast in the role of gods. They seldom mind if patients see other doctors for second opinions. If a doctor does mind, it may be time to consider changing physicians.

Finally, Judy got informed by reading. She read newspaper articles and research studies. She looked at what was written about mastectomies and lumpectomies. Then she made an informed choice. Of course, not all of us can do that because our decision may have to be made more quickly in an emergency situation, or we may not have the ability or strength to do such research. But usually we can find someone who has done the research and can summarize information for us.

No One Cares More about Your Health than You Do

This book is about taking an active approach to health. This may sound very new to some people. We are taught in society and often in our churches that we are victims of disease, that illness is something that happens to us over which we have no control. I do not deny here that the ultimate control is not ours. That is in the hands of Someone greater than ourselves. But we have been given the tools to take a more positive approach to health care and thereby perhaps to live out the joyous life that was intended for us.

This book grew out of nine years of research in which I studied how cancer patients responded when they practiced the healing principles summarized in this book. In that study we found that patients who followed these principles were 59 percent more likely to be well at the end of five years than those who did not. We discovered that changing specific areas of lifestyle could increase one's likelihood of getting well and staying well.

Of course we all must die someday, but who made a rule that we have to die sick? My choice is to live a full, high-quality life filled with faith, love, joy, celebration, caring and understanding in spite of occasional pain, and then to die well.

Is preventing disease really a possibility? Can we learn techniques that will help our bodies heal themselves? Is this fact or fantasy? I believe this is fact. We can live longer, happier, and healthier lives. This is preventive medicine.

In 1980 I asked Dr. Burkitt of England why more emphasis was not placed on prevention. He said, "Because we pay more for mopping up water than we do for turning off faucets." Perhaps what I'm offering here are plumbing lessons.

Chapter 2

A True Story Is the Best Story

Some of the people best suited to teach us how to live are those who are dying. The skills I want to teach in this book were gleaned from cancer patients who were given little hope of living. In sharing the following stories, it is not my intention to take pot shots at the medical profession or suggest that patients should substitute these new skills for conventional medical treatment. I do believe, however, that the techniques and skills here can have a positive effect on health.

Most medical professionals I've known—and I've known many—care about their patients and are searching for ways to help them. Usually, their cups of knowledge are not so full that more cannot be poured into them. Many welcome input from psychology and religion. While there are those who reject new input, I cannot condone such a closed attitude.

None of us has the total answer. We are searching together, and one way that we gather information is through the experiences of others. When a patient responds favorably to treatment, responds better than anyone expected, we want to know that story. As we hear these stories, we recognize that the mind and body work together. As we listen to the stories of cancer patients, we begin to find out how.

Dave

Six years ago Dave came into my office. His doctor had diagnosed lung cancer six months earlier and had removed the upper right lobe of Dave's lung. Not many months after his surgery, Dave was informed that the cancer had spread to the stem of his brain.

It was late December when Dave came to see me on a referral by his radiologist. His physician had given him a short life expectancy—perhaps three months at most. His internist and his oncologist had confirmed this prognosis. He urgently needed to get his affairs in order before he became incapacitated.

Understandably, Dave looked terrible. He was thin. He wore a wig. His face was drawn. I asked him why he had come to me.

"I know that you work with cancer patients," he said. "I'm hoping you can help me deal with this situation."

I knew he was talking about the probability of his death. I asked him, "Do you think you are dying?"

"Yes, and I need help in facing it." Dave was obviously resigned to the fact of his death and desirous of handling the necessary details. I was amazed at his ability to talk about his death in such a matter-of-fact manner and with so much control. I didn't think my own reaction, in his place, would have been so calm, but none of us knows how we will react until we face such a reality.

"Do you want to work on getting well?" was my next question. With experience, I've discovered that people rarely answer this question with an automatic "yes." Many patients have decided far in advance of treatment that they are tired of living. Some have already chosen to die, at least on a subconscious level. But there are others with a dogged determination to live. And even when patients give this question a clear, determined reply, they sometimes change their minds later on.

Dave was genuinely surprised to be asked. "I didn't know I had that choice," he answered, knowing the confirmed prognosis of his cancer.

"Of course you do." I paused, looking for words that would be positive but would still maintain integrity. "There are no guarantees, but it can happen. You might get well, and I'm willing to help you in any way that I can."

Dave could see that I really meant what I said. The commitment I was making to help him enabled him to begin to trust. Therapists and physicians seem to get better results when they really care about their patients—when they love them. This feeling cannot be faked, but if it is real, the patient's trust grows.

Positive thinking. Dave needed positive thoughts and people around him. I wanted to feed his mind with every positive thought possible, and the first idea I wanted him to grasp was *hope* for the future. I believe in hope. I honestly believe that it is better to face any trial of life, including death, with a heart filled with hope.

So, one of the first steps Dave and I took toward improving his health was the restructuring of his negative thoughts. This process is called "cognitive restructuring." Dave needed consciously to change his belief system, shifting his ideas from weak and negative to strong and positive. (See step 2 in Chapter 4.)

Stress reduction. The next step was to tackle his stress. Dave learned skills that helped him to relax. This was important because of the known connection between stress and disease. Stress retards the immune system and makes a person more susceptible to all kinds of disease, even cancer. It's a simple jump to reason that removing any hindrance to the immune system would give the body a better chance to fight cancer and win! So Dave and I worked at reducing his stress.

Positive mental pictures. I also encouraged Dave to work with positive imagery. No one knows just how or why this technique seems to work. Professional sports players have been using it for years. It may be that our bodies produce the things we see most clearly in our minds. Most of us don't realize that we continually, every day, often every moment, have images of ourselves. Positive imagery means choosing to envision health and wholeness. Unlike those obsessed with visions of sickness, people who are obsessed with thoughts of wellness tend to be well, or at least have a better chance than those who are focused on disease.

It makes sense to me that what helps us get well could help prevent us from getting sick. So, I encourage people to talk, think, and imagine being healthy. (See Chapter 9.)

Exercise and nutrition. In addition, Dave and I worked up a reasonable exercise plan for him. Within days, he had joined a health club with a three-month membership. Not long after that he changed it to a lifetime membership.

Dave also met with a nutritionist. She unfortunately believed that nutrition was the total solution to all health problems, but she provided Dave with some helpful information about the value of good nutrition. From the nutritionist, Dave gleaned some guidelines for healthy eating that may have added to his energy and his longevity.

Faith in God. Dave also had come to me to talk about his faith in God. Like most people, Dave had a basic faith but wasn't very clear about what he believed. A clear personal faith brings a sense of security and peace that further reduces stress and frees the body to use its healing system.

Tragically, there are many medical professionals who are reluctant to discuss faith with patients, especially if they are in public health-care settings. Yet, without promoting our own religious viewpoint, those of us in the medical professions can still give spiritual support to those who need it. Very ill people naturally think about the end of life and what that means. More than once I have been asked by a cancer patient to teach him or her how to pray. I'm happy to give that kind of support, and most hospitals do not try to prevent staff from doing so.

Personal faith, in my opinion Christian faith, alleviates fears of death and concerns with guilt. Personalized faith can energize us and enable us to rest more peacefully. We should always feel free to talk about and ask about faith. Dave did.

Dave worked diligently in all the areas we talked about. He became more open about his feelings. He scheduled more fun into his life by going to hockey games, taking trips with his wife, and skiing. Dave practiced relaxation and imagery at least three times every day by listening to a relaxation tape, and he changed his internal belief system by deliberately replacing negative thoughts with positive ones. He clarified his faith by moving from a general, impersonal faith to a specifically Christian, personal faith in a personal God. Dave improved his diet, adding fiber from fruits and vegetables, and he exercised regularly.

In three months, Dave was not in a coma. He and his wife were skiing in Aspen, Colorado! By midsummer they were vacationing in New England. (They sent me a can of pure maple syrup as a memento of that trip.)

A year later, Dave was fighting a recurrence. Fluid had collected in his lungs. That was removed, and Dave took massive doses of chemotherapy for the metastasis (spreading) of cancer into his right hip. One morning after he had received a massive dose of chemotherapy, I called his home and asked him how the treatment was going.

He said, "Anyone who had bet I'd be sick would have lost money. My wife, my son and I are going to see the Blues play hockey tonight."

That answer typified Dave's reactions at that time in his life. He consistently responded to treatment better than expected.

Two years later there was a recurrence that was not diagnosed until the pressure on his brain stem had paralyzed him. Dave died at home. His wife later told me that she and Dave believed that the program he and I had put together for him had added quality and time to his life. She said, "Thank you for the additional time you helped us enjoy."

Dave turned a corner when he found hope for the future. Early on in our work together, he told me, "You have given me hope!"

Best of all, Dave discovered this important truth: "People stand a better chance of being healthy, getting well, or preventing disease if they participate in their own health care; if they help themselves."

Ann

When Ann, a thirty-four-year-old cancer patient, first came to my office, she was in a state of total despair and fatigue. If not consciously, she had at least decided unconsciously that she wanted to die. One of her breasts had been removed surgically, and now cancer had entered her lymph system.

At one point we discussed reconstructive surgery. "I thought about it," she told me, "but there's no point." Ann believed she was dying, and it seemed as if she didn't care.

There are many reasons people opt to die. They may find responsibilities or pain too much to endure. Some feel trapped in a miserable marriage or dead-end job. Death is at least a way out. Often people feel guilty about some real or imaginary sin, and with no sense of a forgiving God, they conclude that they "deserve" to die. Others believe that, having failed in some endeavor and fearing humiliation, they could "just die!"

When people decide to die, whether consciously or unconsciously, there is little that can be done for them. In Ann's case, the challenge was to equip her with skills to help her participate in her own recovery and treatment and also to help her face the reality of the choice she made.

Ann went through a soul-searching struggle and consciously made the decision to live. She has questioned that decision a few times but still seems clear in her commitment to live as well and as long as she can. Now, after successful reconstructive surgery, her life is happier than it has ever been. Ann no longer sees herself as powerless and victimized.

Ann is finding useful activities for herself and is consciously seeking to deepen her personal faith. When Ann discovered her worth and value to God as a person with purpose and a right to express her feelings, she experienced a growing sense of peace and strength.

Ann has adopted a nutritional diet with lower fat and higher fiber foods. The woman who once felt despair now practices relaxation and imagery and has exchanged many of her negative thoughts for more realistic and positive ones. However long Ann's life may be, it will be a life of higher quality than she has ever known before. Ann is living! Ann has hope.

Is Death Failure?

There are other true stories from my experience with cancer patients—some happy, some sad. Some of the patients with whom I have worked have died. Others have extended their lives, and some are cancer-free.

I remember I was greatly disappointed when a certain lady with whom I had worked for about two years died. I told her oncologist, "I feel as though we failed her."

"Not by a long shot," he replied. "When we got her, she was dying of lung cancer. Her life expectancy was less than three months." He asked me if I remembered what she had asked of us.

I did.

"She wanted to live to see her youngest son married and to see her oldest son graduate from one of the Ivy League schools in two years," the oncologist went on. "She saw it all and even the birth of a grandchild. She died happily and peacefully. We did not fail her."

I realized he was right. This woman had put to use all the skills we taught her, and she lived until her goals were reached.

Of course if I had my way, everyone would live and remain healthy. Even as a Christian it's a hard concept for me to accept that sometimes death is a friend. Still I fight for life. I always fight for life.

Of all the patients who worked in our program, a program designed to assist cancer patients, not even one failed to live longer than the average for his or her cancer.

Clint

Clint was a warm and likable, African-American jazz drummer. When I first met him, he weighed 140 pounds; he was very thin for a man nearly six feet tall. He had given up on life and had just rented a room in a local hotel, intending to die there. A professional baseball player who knew me from my team associations saw him at the hotel and suggested that he come to see me and work in the cancer program.

Clint had what I call "sad eyes." They were empty-looking and told of all the weariness from personal struggles Clint was experiencing. There was no trace of humor on his face. Part of his painful past included a recent divorce. And now Clint was afraid he wouldn't be able to get his daughter into medical school, a dream he shared with her.

At first the only energy he showed was when we spoke of the possibility of reuniting his family. Clint and I worked together to restructure Clint's negative thoughts, to replace despair with hope. Best of all, we started having fun together. We told funny stories to each other, went out to eat, and even shot baskets.

Clint seemed to enjoy the genuine acceptance and love he received from our program staff. There were many days that he would just visit at the office and even take a nap in one of the spare rooms. "I just like being here," he explained.

This previously humorless man developed an infectious laugh! Clint laughed, relaxed, and worked his way back to health. Within six months he weighed 178 pounds and had returned to work, playing jazz drum. For five years, I enjoyed Clint's friendship. During that time, Clint spent wonderful times with his family, and he reached his dream of seeing his daughter in medical school.

Then Clint died. I'll never know the "why" of his death, but I do know that purpose and faith and hope gave him several good years he wouldn't have had otherwise.

Vita

There was a patient with Hodgkins disease whose life has been a magnificent example of strength and inspiration for more than fourteen years now. Vita remains cancer-free, as do many Hodgkins patients, but her story is especially remarkable because Vita is a singer, and radiation had damaged her vocal chords.

Vita was a vivacious twenty-one-year-old whom I met when I was doing research at a hospital on the effects of lifestyle changes on cancer. She was diagnosed with "Stage II Hodgkins." Stage I is the least serious, and stage IV the most critical.

Vita's outward attitude was flippant, but that was only a cover for some very serious concerns and fears. Her father had died about two years before Vita discovered her own illness. It has often been documented that one of the conditions that precedes the onset of cancer is the experience of a serious loss in the patient's life (LaShan, *You Can Fight for Your Life*). Perhaps such losses and the ensuing grief create so much stress that the immune system is retarded and unable to fight disease, even cancer. (But there's hope as the principles in this book offer ways to reduce stress and so revitalize the immune system.)

When I approached Vita about our research project, she was in the waiting room at the radiology center. She thought about it for a minute and then with apparent disdain said, "Oh, ___, I'll help you with your study."

Vita became part of our experimental group—the group with which I worked to make lifestyle changes and later compared to a control group that did not receive any interventions. This meant that Vita practiced stress reduction with a relaxation tape and imaging.

Vita was an independent and delightful person, as may be seen in her written report: "I use my own method of relaxation, and I use visualization every night unless I'm so pooped that I drop dead at the sight of a pillow. After visualizing I feel much more in control and am able to fall asleep without dwelling on any problems."

Vita used the process of imaging until she became, in her words, "a Mohammed Ali in my fight against cancer." She then employed the same process of imagery in her fight to regain the use of her vocal chords and larynx. Vita's doctors had told her she would never be able to sing again. Now she is not only cancer-free, but she can once again belt out songs with the best of them.

What about Your Story?

I have briefly told the stories of Dave, Ann, Clint, and Vita to show how each of them became involved positively in his/her own health care. The attitudes and skills that either saved or prolonged their lives, I believe, can help prevent disease as well as cure it.

You can be part of your own health care in the same ways. Keep the following list before you, and commit to make these improvements in your health and lifestyle.

1. *Clarify your purpose for living.* Set goals. We all do better with our lives if we have a "why"!
2. *Clarify your faith*—not in a spiritual being who will exercise total control over you, but in One who will love and empower you to work for your own health and well-being. Choose the path of peace and love.
3. *Seek avenues for spiritual cleansing* from bitterness or unforgiveness. Those ugly twins can drain your energy and make you sick.
4. *Choose joy in life.* Enjoying life is the best reason for living. Have some fun.
5. *Develop relaxation skills* and use them daily.
6. *Remember to really breathe!* Take at least eight to ten deep breaths three times a day or do regular aerobic exercise.
7. *Use your imagination to help you.* Picture reaching your goal of good health and your immune system successfully fighting all disease.
8. *Restructure your negative belief systems.* Think positively and realistically.
9. *Begin a regular, common-sense exercise program.*
10. *Use good judgment in your diet.* Eat plenty of fiber and fruit and vegetables. Avoid excessive fat.

Why do you want to get well or stay well?

A few years ago, I was in a group addressed by Dr. Lawrence LaShan. He told us that when we get sick it is as if our immune systems look up at us and say, "Why should we work to help you get well?" LaShan said that when the only answers we have to give are "I have so much to do. I have duties to fulfill. I have too much responsibility to be sick," then our immune systems kick back and take a rest while we figure out a better answer.

The right answer to the question is "Because I enjoy living." That kind of answer makes our immune systems work a lot harder for us.

When the risk of death seems preferable to changing unhealthy life patterns, some people choose to die. One businessman with bladder cancer was a good example of this fact. He went on a stress reduction program. He lightened his schedule, relaxed, and began an exercise program. The tumor on his bladder shrunk.

But he came to my office one day and said, "I know that if I continue this reduced schedule, I can probably get well and live a long time, but this is just not living for me. I am going back to a heavier work schedule. I love the stress."

He resumed his former way of life, and the tumor grew again. Was it a coincidence? All I know is that he died within three months.

So make your choice for life, and stick by it. Because, after all, it is a choice. We can choose hope, purpose, and power. We choose to become active participants in our own health care. We choose to take the steps to health and wholeness. We choose life!

Chapter 3

Step One: Choose to Live!

The very first step toward health and wholeness is making the choice to live.

Usually, when I make that statement, the first thing people say is, "What? Living is not a choice." I bypass this common reaction by asking them to keep an open mind as we try to learn together.

People often don't see life as a choice because they've stopped looking for choices. One of the most difficult problems I encounter in counseling is the sense of discouragement and despair in the lives of patients. I've found that many people feel like victims. Life just happens to them. Victims make few decisions because they feel helpless.

But there are choices we can make that move us toward living—choices that change the direction of our lives, choices that make us active participants in our own health and wholeness, choices that empower us.

Choose to Participate

The first choice that takes us toward life—or health and wholeness—is the decision to become an active participant in our own health programs. The choice is yours, even if you are presently ill. If you are ill, the decision to participate actively in your health care can give you a better chance of becoming well again. If you are currently healthy, this decision certainly gives you a better chance of staying free of disease.

Being a participant is simply choosing to become active—to do whatever it takes to make yourself a healthier person. "Healthy" can mean different things to different people, but for all of us it means a commitment to seeking alternatives and gathering information. We are empowered by alternatives and action plans.

My friend Rex told me he dreamed he was surrounded by a mob of hostile people intent on doing him bodily harm. But he wasn't worried, because he also dreamed he had a gun. His only problem was that the gun wouldn't fire, no matter how he tried.

You probably know how he felt dreaming such a dream. Most of us have had similar dreams in which we try to scream but no sound comes out.

Rex's dream took place just after he had been diagnosed with cancer. He was feeling helpless; his dream reflected that he felt like a victim. As we talked about the options available to him, Rex began to feel the power of choice. He saw that there were things he could do for himself—many of the things we'll discuss in this book. His options helped activate him, and he became a participant.

When I saw Rex three weeks later, he was beaming, "I dreamed the same dream last week, but this time the gun fired!"

Simply having choices energizes us and provides a sense of power. Recognizing our choices is the beginning of excellence.

Choose to Live

If I asked you, "Do you really want to live?" you'd probably respond by saying, "Are you kidding? Doesn't everybody?" Actually, no. Not everyone wants to live. People who are in tremendous pain, people who feel trapped by life, people who are depressed, and those who are generally discouraged about the future may have no real desire to live. Often they have not made this decision consciously, although there are a few who openly reject life.

When Sue walked into my office and sat in the brown chair across from the couch, I was delighted to see that she seemed to be in a good mood. I knew she was a cancer patient, and I was encouraged by her happiness, thinking it could be a sign that she was developing a positive attitude toward life in spite of her cancer.

It didn't take me long to find out I was completely wrong. I asked Sue how she felt when she was diagnosed.

"I felt like I had been given a reprieve," she told me. "Now I won't have to kill myself; the cancer will do it for me." Sue did not want to live. Sue felt trapped by life. She'd been divorced and was working at a job with a harsh and insensitive supervisor, and she felt she was too old to start a new career.

I wanted to help Sue discover her alternatives. Once she realized that going on permanent disability meant she would never have to go back to that job, she got interested in her future. She decided to work on her own health care—and that was a decision to live.

Stop and think about it. Do you love life? Do you really want to live? Then make the decision. Say it out loud to yourself, "Here and now, I consciously choose to live." Say it again and again: "I choose to live."

Choose to Drop Bad Habits

More and more the medical community is discovering that lifestyle is the major predictor of good or poor health. An instructor in "wellness" from the University of Missouri says that the combination of genetic inheritance, environment, and health-care systems account for about forty-nine percent and that fifty-one percent of personal health is the result of lifestyle. If she's right, more than fifty percent of your health depends on the choices you make! So choose to avoid the unhealthy lifestyle options of smoking, abusing alcohol or other drugs, living with high levels of stress, refusing to deal honestly with emotions, eating junk foods, withdrawing from people in fear, and feeding on negative self-talk (the things we say to ourselves in our minds).

My favorite definition of insanity is, "Insanity is doing the same thing, the same way, over and over again, but expecting the results to change." If you want different results, you must change what you are doing.

I smoked for many years, even after I knew how much damage it could do to my system. Knowing it was bad for me didn't change anything. I was really hooked. At least that was my excuse until I made the decision to give myself the gift of fresh air. I made a conscious choice to live, and that meant I would immediately stop smoking.

You can drop your bad habits.

Choose to Be Responsible

My grandmother used to say, "Every tub sits on its own bottom." It was her way of saying that each person is responsible for himself or herself. This is a difficult lesson for many people to learn, but it is a healthy lesson.

It's a common pastime to play the "blame game." Too many of us go through life blaming someone or something for our problems. "I can't because . . . my father was Irish, German, African, English, poor, uneducated, alcoholic, or whatever." "I can't because I'm . . . [fill in the blank: too old, too young, too tired, too sick, too dumb, a man, a woman, a White person, an African-American, etc.]"

Forget the blame game. The truth is that you're responsible for yourself—for your attitudes, your behavior, your anger, your happiness, and much of your health. But even this responsibility is a choice. When you accept the responsibility, it means you've got to change your language. Compare these statements by "victims" and by responsible participants.

Step One: Choose to Live!

Victims	Participants
I must.	I choose.
That's just the way I am.	I can be different.
She makes me mad.	I got mad.
I should.	It would be better.
I can't.	I don't want to.
If only.	I will.
They won't let me.	I choose not to.
I am a victim.	I am a participant.
It's not my fault.	I accept responsibility.

If the list on the left looks a little too familiar, clean up your language and become an active participant in your own life.

A few years ago I was complaining that I had too much to do. Probably I was just looking for sympathy or at least an admiring, "I don't see how you do it." But my friend wouldn't give me what I expected; instead she gave me what I needed.

"Who makes your schedule?" she asked, knowing that, of course, I did.

I have another friend who has a late-night radio show. When callers tell Jim to "Have a nice day," he responds, "I'll have any kind of day I want!"

It may not be polite, but Jim's answer is right. Each person, at least to some significant degree, determines the kind of day—or life—to have. The choice belongs to us.

Choose to Exercise Your Rights

I often tell people that I believe we all have at least three basic rights.

First, you have the right to take what is and make the most of it. You can take a look at your situation and do your best with it. Some people do this without complaining. They focus on what they *can* do, not on what they cannot do. They're making a positive choice.

Next, you have the right to have as much fun as you can in life. In chapter 8, we'll talk more about having fun and celebrating life. Look for ways to have fun; it'll make a difference in how you feel.

Finally, you have the right to leave your own "thumbprint" on this world. None of us is like anyone else, and each of our personalities are valid. No one can do what you can do in this world. Will you do it? The choice is yours.

It's Personal

Will you choose to live and to live well? You can do it. It's your personal choice. Henry David Thoreau, the American philosopher and writer, said: "I know of no more encouraging fact than the unquestionable ability of man to elevate his life by conscious endeavor." Although we may disagree with some of what Thoreau stood for, we can learn from his ability to live each day to its fullest. And who can be our primary model of someone who lived each day full of meaning and purpose? Christ. We can learn from him how to celebrate the life God has given us, even when that life may be short.

Participating This Week

In appendix A you will find seven meditations. During the next week, read one each day and then record your thoughts about it in your own notebook. You may want to refer back to this chapter and see if the concepts are becoming clearer for you.

Chapter 4

Step Two: Adopt Healthy Beliefs

People throw around the phrase "quality of life" until it has little meaning. What constitutes "quality" is arbitrary—different for each person.

A person's quality of *health* is also a personal thing. It is largely determined by each person's internal belief system. Those internal beliefs are vastly important to each person's physical well-being. Mind and body cannot be separated—and beliefs and health can't be parted either.

The mind-body system is something like a fabulously intricate computer. A lot of people don't realize that data is constantly being put into their "computers." Their minds are continuously processing their experiences. Everything they see, hear, think, or feel—positive or negative—goes into their minds. And everything that goes in will have some effect, even if years go by before we see the end results.

How Beliefs Influence Behavior

One of my own idiosyncrasies demonstrates the power of "input." Until recently, I had difficulty buying shoes. For some reason I always thought, "This pair will last a little longer," or "I'm sure I can find a cheaper pair." Even when I purchased shoes at a cut-rate store, on sale, I'd still feel guilty. Why? Because the data (beliefs) put into my computer (my mind) were putting out guilt.

Then I realized where those beliefs originated. My parents had little money while I was growing up, so they told me repeatedly, "Take care of your shoes. If you are just going to play, go barefoot, and save your shoes for school or Sunday." Our family half-soled shoes, put heels on them, and put taps on the heels and toes. My parents admonished my siblings and me not to "roll our shoes over" or stand on the sides of them because we "couldn't afford to buy new shoes." I never consciously decided, "I will always be careful about buying new shoes," but I was unconsciously influenced by all those admonitions and experiences.

Money wasn't my problem. I could've purchased a vacation ticket to Athens, Greece, without feeling guilty—even though the ticket price would buy a lot of very nice shoes. I didn't have data in my computer prohibiting that kind of purchase!

What I heard as a child was still influencing me forty years later. I had to identify those erroneous and negative beliefs, change them, and act on my new beliefs. Now, of course, I've successfully worked to overcome that sense of guilt. I've changed my beliefs and acted on my new beliefs—in this case, buying new shoes!

Whatever goes into your mind will have an effect on you. Your own self-talk affects your attitudes and health. In his "Mind Revolution" seminars, I have heard Anthony Robbins say, "The quality of your life is the quality of your communication to yourself and others." So what does it mean to communicate to yourself? Whether you know it or not, you're "self-talking" all the time.

No matter what we do, our minds will register experience. We can't control whether or not our minds will record mental input, but we can control what that input will be. We can deliberately, consciously decide which thoughts to put into our minds.

Think of your mind as a tree and thoughts as birds. You can't stop a bird from flying in and perching in your tree, but maybe you can determine which birds build nests and stay.

Prisms of Perception

Beliefs form what I like to call "prisms of perception." These prisms become filters for our experiences. The same experience may happen to two different people, but they will view it in different ways because they filter it through different prisms.

If you want to change your interpretations and reactions to life, change your beliefs. For example, I believe that life is usually *fun,* but I know a man who believes that life is usually *miserable*. Recently I was forgotten by a friend who was going to take me to lunch while I was in Ft. Lauderdale, Florida. I reacted to that experience according to my prism of perception. I looked around for a way to have fun, despite my unfortunate situation. I wound up crashing a buffet luncheon and meeting some very nice people. It was a fun day.

In the same situation, my friend who believes life is generally miserable would probably have sat in the hotel bemoaning the fact that he was "born to lose" (the title of one of his favorite songs).

A person's reaction is a result not only of the experience, but of the perception or belief through which the experience is filtered.

Adopting New Beliefs

If mind influences body, then it stands to reason that we are doing ourselves a favor when we put healthy, positive thoughts into our minds. These positive perceptions can help us prevent or overcome disease. One way to incorporate such positive thoughts is to find out what healthy people's perceptions are and adopt them as our own.

To make a belief your own, you must be open to recognizing possibilities and desire to believe. Four simple—but not easy—steps can help you adopt new beliefs.

First, identify any negative belief you want to change. State it in order to see it clearly. Then, reshape that belief in honest and realistic positive terms.

Suppose, for example, you want to change the belief that you aren't a popular person. State your negative belief clearly: "I don't have any friends." Then express the same idea in constructive terms: "Although I don't have as many friends as I would like to have, I do have some friends and I can gain more each month."

Anyone would feel better believing the second statement! Work to reshape negative beliefs into healthier and more positive ideas.

Next, entrench that new belief in your mind. You've found a positive way to look at a problem, so repeat that positive statement. Write out the positive concept and commit an exact wording to memory. Say it out loud. Tell someone else. Say it again and again. Repeat the belief to yourself until it is firmly entrenched in your mind.

Then, each time you find yourself reverting to the old, negative way of thinking about that problem, correct your thought. To continue our example, suppose someone came up to you and said, "Gee, you sure don't have many friends." You should immediately correct that person: "I don't have as many as I'd like, but I do have some, and I'm making new friends all the time."

Don't kid yourself. Permanent change is not easy to effect. Desire alone won't bring permanent change. Just reading this book won't accomplish it, either. It will come after weeks, even months of work, but change is worth the effort when it raises the quality of your life and health.

The third step is to picture your life the way you'd like it to be. At the same time that you're changing the way you talk to yourself and others about your problem, imagine your life the way you would like it to be. Picture yourself enjoying new friends and seeing old ones socially. In your imagination, hear someone say, "You sure seem to be making a lot of friends."

Keep imagining such an idea until it becomes a real possibility in your mind. Repeat it until you believe that it is possible. Repeat it until you believe that it is

Step Two: Adopt Healthy Beliefs

probable. Repeat it until you believe it. Repeat it until it becomes a conviction. Repeat it until you know that it is true. Perhaps you think this is just creating a delusion. But I believe it is creating a self-fulfilling prophecy.

As you see that you've adopted a new belief, you'll find yourself practicing the new technique in other situations. For example, one negative thought would be: "If she leaves me, I'll never be happy. I'll always be alone and abandoned." The positive take is: "It will be painful if she leaves me, but it will not be the end. There are other relationships. I will make it, and I will be happy." According to the process, you'd repeat that positive statement and refuse any negative input. You'd imagine yourself standing strong and hear yourself saying, "I knew I could be happy on my own."

This works for those who are ill as well. The negative thought might go like this: "I am sick. I have cancer (or heart disease, or whatever illness troubles you). I am going to die." The positive phrasing would be: "Of course, I'm sick, but I can get well. Other people have overcome this disease. So can I. I will die someday, as everyone does, but I might not die of cancer. My body will do what it takes to heal itself." Then repeat it until you know it is true.

One cancer patient told me, "I used to say I'd get well, but wonder whether or not I would. I just said it because I wanted to believe it. Now I do believe it. I know it. I am going to get well." He had lung cancer, with metastases to the brain and bone. He overcame the nausea he was experiencing with chemotherapy. Now his brain scan is clear, and he seems to be getting well.

Repetition helps you climb the steps—from possibility to probability to belief to conviction, right up to knowing. Climb these stairs:

        KNOWLEDGE
        CONVICTION
        BELIEF
        PROBABILITY
        POSSIBILITY

When a belief becomes so ingrained that you "know" it, it then belongs to you, and you will act on it.

Of course, some will point out that there are people who "know" they are getting well and still they die. I have known people who prayed for healing and really believed they were being healed and still they died. I don't understand why that happened, but I would not discourage those people from believing, and I would not discourage people from "knowing" they are getting better. The closer people come to "knowing" that healing is taking place, the more hope and peace they experience, and these are more conducive to health than fear and insecurity.

The fourth step is to act on the new belief. Once you have entrenched a new belief, you can act as if that belief is true.

When I was in college, I read about the philosophy of the German thinker Hans Vaihinger. He based his ideas, which he called Fictional Finalism, on the notion that we all have a belief about life, a fiction that might or might not be true. We then act "as if" that belief were final and always true.

We may believe, for example, that all tall people should be feared. This may be true. But whether it's true or not is irrelevant to our behavior. We act as if it were true and tend to avoid tall people.

Other beliefs are far more important to our lives and health. If I believe that my body is healthy and, within reason, I act on that belief, my thoughts can have a positive effect on my health.

What to Believe

So, what sorts of beliefs will help us be healthy? The following beliefs are healthy, empowering, and life-giving. They are some of the beliefs of healthy people. Some come from people who have survived serious illnesses. Others are from people who seem to be living healthy, happy lives. If you choose to adopt any or all of them, you can. Begin by examining the beliefs. If you like them, write them, memorize them, and begin repeating them to yourself.

Healing power. Healthy belief number one: "There is healing power in me. My body is working for me. My body is working to fight disease and make me healthy."

There is no way to know how much effect our internal beliefs have on our health, but we theorize that negative thoughts, fear, and expectation of illness certainly do not and cannot help us. Unfortunately, that's not always the message we give or get. We tend to teach and learn unhealthy beliefs about health.

For example, when a child goes outside in cold weather, parents often comment: "If you get cold, you'll get sick." "If you get your feet wet, you'll get sick." Other common statements describe negative beliefs about the body's power to fight illness. "This awful flu is really going around. If you haven't caught it yet, it won't be long." (I never understood the use of the word *caught* to refer to illness. If I'm not chasing illness I won't "catch" it.)

When was the last time you heard, "If you get cold, try to find a place to get warm. But don't worry. Your body is strong and fights disease really well"? And who says to you, "Sure, there's a lot of sickness going around, but you're strong and healthy. You rarely get sick." Even if no one else gives you such positive input, you can give it to yourself. If you are a cancer patient, adopt this positive belief: "My body is working to fight cancer. My body will do whatever it takes to help me get well." Phrase it any way you like, but make it healthy.

There is a proverb: "The mind and body talk to each other, and the conversation is often fatal." It doesn't have to be. Keep on talking to yourself with life-giving, empowering conversation.

Worth and value. Healthy belief number two: "My life is worth living. I have as much right to live as anyone. I don't have to prove my worth and value. Worth and value are mine because I am a human being: God gives my life value, and no one can take it away."

These are sentences to commit to memory. Your self-image is one of your most important assets—or a liability. If you believe in your own worth and value, there is little that you cannot achieve, including better

Step Two: Adopt Healthy Beliefs

health. Remember this: "No one lives life consistently at a level inconsistent with his or her self-concept or self-image."

You live according to your own "fictions" about life. Your belief about your abilities determines the level of your achievement. I've seen this to be true in my experience. When I was working as a team psychologist for the St. Louis Cardinals from 1980-1982, I saw a clear demonstration of the power of self-image on performance. Player Keith Hernandez told me many times that he was a .300 hitter. If he was hitting at the .240 level, and I asked him what he thought he would hit for the season, he'd reply, "Three hundred." Guess what his lifetime average is? .300. People perform at a level consistent with their beliefs about themselves.

Another baseball player offers an even more dramatic example. Phil Bradley was formerly with the Seattle Mariners, and I was their team psychologist from 1983–1987. Phil hit one home run in his first full season in the major leagues, but in his second season he hit twenty-six home runs. Talk about major improvement! I asked Phil what made the difference. He told me, "No one ever told me I could hit home runs before this year." Hitting coach Daren Johnson had told him that he could do it. Bradley believed it, and he did it.

Believing you can achieve doesn't work only in baseball; it also will work in your everyday life. People perform at levels consistent with their self-beliefs.

So what does your self-image have to do with your physical health? People who believe they have worth and value behave as if they do. But those who doubt their worth become discouraged, and discouragement often leads to despair. And despair often leads to sickness.

I once met a woman who was abusing her body with drugs. She knew it was bad for her, and she seemed to be sorry about it, but she was convinced she couldn't stop. However, she did stop. She told me that what helped her put an end to her drug abuse was finding out she was a person of value. She said, "You told me I was better than that. I was worth saving. I could expect better things of myself than drug abuse. I had never thought about my drug abuse having anything to do with my value, but it does. I won't use drugs again." And she hasn't.

God thought so much of the value of human beings that "he gave his one and only Son, that whoever believes in him shall not perish but have eternal life" (John 3:16).

Wouldn't it be great to eliminate a great deal of discouragement? We could do it by helping people recognize their worth. Those who believe in themselves are filled with courage and hope, and that makes them healthier, more productive people.

Self-concept is crucial. Commit yourself to improving yours now. Beliefs can change, and when they do behavior and life change, too. There are several practical things you can do to help improve your self-esteem.

1. No one can make you think less of yourself unless you permit it. Make up your mind not to let anyone reduce your view of yourself.
2. Read good, encouraging material. There are plenty of books designed to help you improve your self-concept. You can also choose to spend

time in good devotional and inspirational works. Self-improvement cassette tapes or videos might also be helpful.
3. Treat yourself as if you have value. Dress up. Buy yourself a healthful meal. Treat yourself to a trip. Just treat yourself in general as if you deserve good things. And take care of your health. You are worth it!
4. Spend time with people who are positive and encouraging. Some people will drag you down. Stay away from them! Seek out people who excite and energize you. Talk with them. Pick their brains, so to speak. Imitate the lifestyle and beliefs of those you admire. If you want to stay healthy, hang out with healthy people and learn to live as they live.

Remember, you have as much worth and value as anyone. Believe it and act as if it is true. You will improve the quality of your life and health by improving your self-concept.

Purpose and meaning. Healthy belief number three: "I have purpose. My life has meaning." You'll find it's easy to believe your life has purpose and meaning when you act as if it has! One practical way to do this is to set some realistic goals for yourself. Make a list of what you want to do. Look closely at your values and beliefs. What do they say about the purpose of your life? Do you have a guiding principle for life? The Westminster Confession gives as the first goal of life for Christians: "To glorify God and enjoy him forever." What is your goal? And what are your short-term goals? Be specific and set goals to achieve in one year, two years, five years, and so on.

Goals have an almost magnetic power. They attract energy and move us in directions that lead to real achievement. Don't be afraid to set goals. Recent health literature indicates that patients without purpose are sicker and die faster than those who have a sense of their reasons for living.

German philosopher and writer Victor Frankl described those who died and those who survived in the concentration camps of World War II, in Germany. Similar descriptions have come from prisoners of war from Korea and Vietnam. People who had a sense of purpose kept their passion for living regardless of the truly evil circumstances around them.

When you have a passion for life, your whole system functions better. Finding meaning is so vital to health that it makes up one of the eight steps toward health listed in this book. We'll talk about it in depth in the following chapter.

For now, let's focus on goal-setting. If you are sick, set a goal for getting well. A patient told me recently, "My goal is to be cancer-free in two years." She thought about how she would look and feel in two years. It was a realistic goal. I do not know if she reached that goal, but I know she was feeling better because of it.

Personally, I have a goal to play basketball well into my retirement years. I've got to be healthy to do that, so exercise and healthy habits are part of my goals.

The old saying goes, "You can't hit what you're not aiming at." Without a goal, you'll never get where you want to be.

All of us set goals on an unconscious level everyday. For example, we rarely set out on a trip without a destination in mind. When was the last time you bought a ticket for a trip and told the ticket agent, "Just give me a ticket for any place"? Choosing a destination for a short trip—or a long one—isn't so different from goal-setting. You're just choosing long-term and short-term goals for where you want to go personally.

Sick people sometimes hesitate to set goals, fearing they won't live to fulfill them. But that's true for all of us. No one has a guarantee on when life will end. My friend, Swoff, used to say, "Plan as if you are going to live forever, and live as if you are going to die today."

Write out or think out some long-term and short-term destinations for yourself. Make a list of what kind of person you want to be, where you want to be, what kind of relationships you want to have, and what kind of health you want to have. Go over that list and designate some as short-term and some as long-term goals. Set goals for one year, two years, five years, a lifetime.

If you find your goals are too vague or general, try to make them specific or measurable. Don't say, "I want to lose weight." But say, "I want to lose fifteen pounds within the next two months."

I started setting goals when I was in junior high school. Because I had good self-esteem I was not reluctant to set goals. I even drew pictures of myself achieving some of those goals. The notebook containing those pictures is one of my valued possessions today.

I wanted to be student body president, set basketball scoring records, play the trumpet in the high school band, get a degree from Washington University, and play professional baseball. The only one I didn't reach was playing baseball professionally, but when I was in spring training working with two different major league teams, I thought it was close enough.

We may achieve some things by accident, but that's rare. Most achievements, and especially good health, come because we have planned for them. Begin planning now. Set some goals and let those goals remind you that you have purpose in life. A personal sense of purpose gives you a better chance for healthy living. Your life has purpose. Repeat it. Believe it. Live as if it is true.

Expressing your feelings. Healthy belief number four: "I have the right to express myself." Holding your feelings inside can be unhealthy. This is especially true if you're holding them in because you think you have no right to express them. Feelings are not right or wrong. It's what we do with them that is good or bad. You have a right to express your own feelings.

Some people have held their feelings in for so long that they can't even recognize them any longer. A person recently asked me, "How can I identify what I am feeling? I can't remember ever expressing my feelings." If you have a hard time knowing how you feel, the best way to start is to guess. Say, "I feel _____"—then just fill in the blank. Keep guessing until your guess feels right to you.

Practice identifying and expressing your feelings with a close friend or spouse. Use the phrases "I feel" and "I want." The two most important things someone can know about you is what you feel and what you want. That is especially true when that person loves you. Some good starters are, "I feel lonely, and I want a hug" and "I feel hungry and want something to eat." If you practice on such simple feelings, pretty soon you'll reach down to the deeper ones.

You have a right to express your feelings. Do it for your health's sake. Repeat it, believe it, and act as if it is true.

Enjoying life. Healthy belief number five: "I enjoy living." The best reason you have for living is that you want to live. You don't need an excuse—you can want to live just because living is fun. A sense of humor and the ability to find delight in everyday things keeps the creative juices flowing—and it's healthy. So be sure to incorporate some fun into your life. Fun is so important that it's another one of the eight steps to good health.

Obviously, not everything in life is fun. But even when things are difficult, you can usually find some level of pleasure. It depends on how you talk to yourself and what you believe about your circumstances.

Every day can be a celebration when you make the decision to take what you have, wherever you are, and make the most of it. Determine not to waste valuable time complaining, which can take away your joy. Focus your attention on the good and humorous things in your life.

Finding hope. Healthy belief number six: "I have hope. If anyone can make it, I can." In a counseling situation, often the best thing I can do for a person is help restore his or her hope.

Hope depends quite a bit on the way you choose to see. Take statistics, for example. If there's a 90 percent chance of rain, there is a 10 percent chance of sunshine! People tend to say, "Well, with that disease, nine out of ten die." Why not phrase it positively? "One in ten lives. I might as well be that one." If everyone approached statistics from a hopeful vantage point, we'd soon change the statistics.

There are few, if any, diseases from which someone has not recovered. Recovery is *always* a possibility. It is also true that there has never been a disease that infected everyone who came in contact with it. In other words, prevention is always possible, and recovery is almost always possible.

I've grounded my life in hope. I hope for cures. I hope for prevention. I hope for better life. Hope is real. In my view, there is no such thing as false hope. Be realistic, but never be afraid to hope. Say, "I have hope." Repeat it, believe it, and live as if it is true.

Whatever it takes. Healthy belief number seven: "I will do whatever it takes. My body will do whatever it takes to fight disease." This statement goes beyond belief—all the way to commitment. Committing to do whatever it takes is a way of life. I will do whatever it takes to be creative, to get well, to accomplish whatever it is that I really want in life, to serve my Creator. I will do whatever it takes, short of hurting others in the process.

Believing you'll do whatever it takes raises your quality of life and health. Commit to it: "I will do whatever it takes." Repeat it, believe it, and live as if it is true.

Be a participant. Healthy belief number eight: "I am in charge of my own life. I am not a victim. I am a participant. I will ask questions. I will put my own thumbprint on this world." Becoming a participant clearly involves personal responsibility. The words "personal responsibility" may be unpopular, but responsibility is healthy. Consider the alternative. You are either responsible or a victim. Repeat this: "I believe I am responsible." Believe it, and act as if it is true.

Accepting responsibility is one of the specific topics for meditation for this chapter. If you do not use those meditations to strengthen your resolve to become healthier, guess who is responsible?

Positive people. Healthy belief number nine: "I am a positive person. I do healthy things and think healthy thoughts." People who reject healthy thinking and actions tend to spiral downward, as poor choices actually become a habit. One man told me in a counseling session, "Even when I can have good things, I keep choosing bad things. I am tearing up my car," he added, "because I keep on driving over the same potholes every day."

A lady told me she was terribly lonely. She said, "I don't answer my phone because the only time it rings is when it is a wrong number."

To a positive person, the answers are obvious. Stop driving over those same potholes. Pick up the phone and talk to whoever is calling. But negative thinkers have gotten out of the habit of looking for solutions. They are prejudiced against themselves.

Recently I talked to a group of executives at the top of their corporation. I asked them to list their own positive attributes and share one or two with the group. Out of fifty people, few mentioned anything. The three or four who did mentioned the positives almost apologetically.

Then I asked them to cite some positive qualities of others in the room. They had so many to offer, I had to cut off the responses.

Then I asked them to list their personal weaknesses, or negative things about themselves. Again, they responded quite freely.

This illustration shows the widespread concept that it's okay to be positive about others, but not about oneself. Throw out that idea, and understand this: It is all right to say good things to and about yourself, no matter what anyone has told you about "bragging." I, only half jokingly, say that I like the beatitude, "Blessed are ye if ye toot your own horn, for verily it shall be well tooted." I believe it is healthy to think and say positive things about yourself.

As we discussed early in this chapter, the way to establish a belief is through repetition. Write it, say it, repeat it, think it, and act as if it is true. Go over the beliefs of healthy people and make them your own.

Remember:
The way to establish a belief is through repetition.
The way to establish a belief is through repetition.
The way to establish a belief is through repetition.

Participating This Week

Look in the Appendix for the meditations for Step Two. As you read them, commit to do what it takes to adopt healthy beliefs. And remember, the way to establish a belief is through repetition.

Chapter 5

Step Three: Find Meaning

I sat straight up in bed. It was 2 A.M. and pitch black. The silence of the night was deadly. My heart was pounding and my body was cold with sweat. I was near panic. I had awakened from a terrible dream—I was dying and was being told by a voice (God's, I presumed) that my life had been wasted, that my life had meant absolutely nothing.

I still hate to think about that dream. Few things would amount to greater tragedy than coming to the end of life and realizing that there was no point to it all.

In these days of instant news and fast travel, many people still live in "quiet desperation." Too often, they go through the motions of living but never really live—because they have no sense of purpose or meaning.

Purpose and meaning are essential to life.

Loss of Meaning

When I was in school during the early 1960s, Victor Frankl was predicting that the next major crisis for our world would be "the loss of meaning." This would be especially devastating, he suggested, because the dominating drive in human beings is the "drive to meaning."

Lawrence Lashan captured the same idea when he claimed that before people can mobilize the will to live they "must first have goals in the future" that are important to them *(You Can Fight For Your Life)*.

The experience of a cancer patient named Julia illustrates in living color the awesome power of goals. She was one of the first cancer patients with whom I worked—a soft-spoken, pleasant woman in her early fifties. She had small-cell carcinoma of the lungs and had been told that her life expectancy was three to six months. I first saw her five months after that diagnosis.

Right away Julia informed me that she could not die yet because she had some very important things to do. Her youngest son's marriage was six months away, and Julia fully intended to be present at the wedding. Julia worked with relaxation, imaging, exercise, and continued her medical treatment. She had a distinct purpose, and it gave her the motivation and energy—the will—to fight for her life.

She attended that wedding!

Then, she told me, her older, married son was expecting a child. Obviously, Julia couldn't die until she saw her first grandchild. She held that child in her arms.

Within a few weeks after that baby's first birthday, Julia was back in the hospital with a recurrence of cancer. I thought she might make it if she could find another purpose for living. "Is there anything else you want to do?" I asked her.

"Not really," Julia told me. She just stared at the ceiling.

Within three weeks, Julia died.

I'd seen Julia's commitments give her courage and strength. If she'd found some purpose that was really important to her, Julia might have lived longer. But when there was no more meaning for her, she gave up her fight.

Looking for Meaning in All the Wrong Places

In this fragmented world, frenzied people are lowering empty buckets into empty wells and pulling them up faster and faster, still empty. They vainly seek meaning, connections, or just anything to fill their lives. The loss of personal security, the loss of personal meaning, the depersonalization of society, work, and medicine have generated a startlingly widespread sense of despair.

One heartbreaking expression of this pervasive problem is that even children sometimes have trouble finding meaning. There was a time when children were needed in their families. They helped with the chores, not as training, but because they were honestly needed. In rural areas, children were a vital part of the family's work unit. Now, in many families, the youngsters often just seem to be in the way. Where will these children find the foundation for their personal meaning?

Another evidence of the desperate clamoring in the absence of meaning is that radical and cultic groups are springing up all over the world. People are searching. They want to belong to something. They want someone or something to give them meaning. Frustrated and desperate people fanatically throw themselves into causes. They do not want to live without a "why."

Saint Augustine wrote that there is a "God-shaped" void in the hearts of people that can never be satisfied until God is welcomed into their lives. It seems clear that this vacuum includes the deep human need for meaning. When we feel detached and meaningless we reach out to whatever is available. We all seem to be crying, "Give me a cause to follow. Give me a reason to live." Maybe we know innately that we need a purpose and that our systems function better when they have a reason to function. People are healthier and more energized with a sense of purpose, a reason for living. Faith gives many people that reason to live. Those who have committed themselves to God and accepted the meaning that Christ offers will find a purpose for living.

Two Levels of Meaning

There exist at least two levels of meaning. There is, in the first place, a philosophical/religious meaning. It is what I call the "Big Picture" or overall level of meaning where we find the answers to questions like,

"What is life?" "Who am I?" and "What is this existence all about?"

People have often told me that they've lived their lives without ever asking those questions, much less answering them. This always surprises me, because I agree with Plato that "the unexamined life is not worth living." And perhaps that's indirectly the point of this book: The unexamined life, or the life without meaning, is frequently an unhealthy life. That's why I believe that religious commitment is a basic ingredient for health.

The second level of meaning holds the less dramatic, seemingly smaller answers for the daily grind. This is the kind of meaning that Julia experienced. She found meaning in immediate goals that were important to her, and that pulled her toward life.

Meaning is vital to me. I believe that my life has purpose, the purpose for which God created me. Purpose means direction; it gives a reason, a "why" I should live. Human beings can endure almost any "how" (circumstance) if they have a "why" (purpose). Think of those who have survived torturous conditions because they were determined to live out a commitment to a cause, their country, or their faith. Meaning provides courage to live and courage to die. It seems to me that meaning also stimulates our immune systems and makes us healthier.

Again, Victor Frankl suggests that since one of the basic psychological forces in life is the drive for meaning to lose that meaning is to lose the will for living.

Make It Happen

Once again, you have to ask, "Am I going to wait for life to happen to me, or am I going to happen to life?"

Those who "happen to life" find meaning and courage to live. But those who wait for life are approaching their days as victims, and they are easily discouraged.

Unfortunately, we've become what Charles Sykes calls "a nation of victims." Far more people are directed by what happens to them than by what happens inside them. We are "outer directed" instead of "inner directed." Circumstances and the opinions of others control us because we've relinquished control by failing to choose our own directions and goals.

Principle-centered people are people of character. These are the strong ones who have the courage to submit themselves to what they believe is right regardless of what society or anyone else says. These people make life happen. They are committed to something or Someone greater than themselves.

If you do not presently have a sense of purpose in life, you can begin to establish direction by setting goals. These don't have to be elaborate goals; they just have to be your own goals. Your goals empower you. You'll find that your goals will pull you along even when you think you've forgotten all about them. Proverbs 29:18 tells us, "Where there is no vision, the people perish" (KJV). God made us people who need goals and purpose to live, and when we have goals our lives are empowered. It's the way we were created.

Inner-Directed Survivors

In my work with cancer patients I have seen some miraculous recoveries. But very few have experienced recovery unless they actively participated in their own health programs. In other words, if they hadn't taken action, exercised, changed their lifestyles, sought meaning, dropped bad habits, took charge of nutrition, and accepted responsibility for themselves, they would not have been as likely to recover from illness or to stay healthy.

I also have seen few recoveries among those without a sense of purpose. Those who recover believe they have a reason to live. Along with countless thousands, I have been inspired by the stories of Dr. Victor Frankl and his experiences in the concentration camps of World War II. I can almost see his emaciated, naked body sitting, hunched forward on the edge of a crude cot. I can picture the resolve and determination never dimming from his eyes, even though he was hungry, tired, and sometimes sick. Frankl would not be beaten. He was inner-directed. The Nazis could beat him, humiliate him, even kill him, but they could never take away his internal freedom to find meaning for himself in his experiences. He survived his ordeal because he found a reason to live.

Take Step Three

Step three is to find purpose for your life. Take that step! Set goals to give you a sense of immediate purpose and long-term meaning. Add to your belief

Step Three: Find Meaning

system, "I have purpose, meaning in my life." Repeat it, believe it, and act as if it is true.

There is tremendous power in affirmation. Author Earl Nightingale said that his greatest discovery was that "we become what we think." In the Bible, Proverbs 23:7 teaches that people become what they think in their hearts. What they think in their hearts is their purpose.

One cancer patient, Lou, told me that for him purpose meant he would leave the world a better place than he found it. Others might have scoffed at Lou's statement; it might have sounded trite to them. But it made sense to Lou, and it helped him.

One morning Lou phoned me shortly after he'd left my office. On his way home, he'd encountered a woman walking beside the highway. Lou saw her many needs, picked her up, purchased some food for her, and rented a motel room for her. He was calling me to see if I could help find a more permanent place for the woman to stay. Lou believes in the purpose he's chosen, and he acts as if it is true.

Lou was onto something—the truth that people find purpose and meaning in alleviating human suffering wherever they find it. You can take part even by doing something as simple as listening to a lonely person, feeding a hungry family, or speaking a word of encouragement to a discouraged person. Meaning and purpose are not necessarily big and dramatic. You can always find a way to mean something to someone else.

You've probably heard before that "God doesn't make junk." He made you, so there is meaning and purpose to your life—the meaning and purpose for which he created you.

Participating This Week

As you identify the meaning and purpose in your own life, the meditations on Step Three, found in appendix A, can be a help and encouragement. Work through them.

Chapter 6

Step Four: Control Stress

What does stress have to do with your health? A lot!

Stress is related to retarding the immune system.
Stress is directly related to heart disease.
Stress is directly related to strokes.
Stress is related to stomach disorders.
Stress is related to accidents.
Stress is related to cancer.
Stress is related to sudden death syndrome.

This list could be even longer, based on the studies of researchers Hans Selye, Carl O. Simonton, Robert Eliot, Thomas Holmes, and Richard Rahe. My own research with cancer patients has also shown stress to be connected to these and other physical problems.

Everyone is subject to stress. Stress is generated by any loss, separation, relocation, new direction, change in health, job change, personal growth, fear, celebration, grief, unrealistic expectation—and many other things.

Stress researchers still usually list work as the most common cause of stress. Among the other top ten stressors are interruptions, managers/supervisors, telephone calls, project assignments, and the family.

Quick Fixes

I recently did a radio call-in program with my friend Jim White. We asked the listeners what they did to relieve stress and got some rather interesting and helpful answers. They may provide some immediate relief from stress, but I recommend that you add a specific stress reduction program to your arsenal of skills for life. These are some of the stress reducers we learned from callers that day:

1. Color pictures in a coloring book. This is a great way to get away from the pressures of the present and for a few minutes be a child again.
2. Play a child's game with or without the help of a child. Just playing can relieve stress.
3. Go out and purchase a toy you always wanted as a child but never received. Play with it!
4. Close your eyes, take a few deep breaths, and imagine you are in a totally white room. If you are having trouble with someone, picture that person there in the room with you as a statue. One caller said that after a few minutes of this, he felt refreshed and relaxed.
5. Take a bath. This was suggested by a mother who said that after she got her two-year-old to

bed, a nice leisurely bath was an immediate stress reliever.

Another good stress reliever is to add variety to your life. Doing the same things in the same way at the same time is likely to push you into a rut. The cure is trying something different. Perhaps the following list will give you some thought starters.

Drive into your driveway in reverse. If you already do this, drive forward. Just do something different.

Write a love note to someone in pig-latin.

Make out a household budget with Roman numerals.

While at lunch, stare through your fork at people and pretend that they are in jail.

Make up a language and use it around the dinner table.

Write a short story using alphabet soup.

You get the idea. Do something that veers off your everyday pattern. It just might provide some short-term stress relief.

Long-range Stress Management

Despite the relief these one-shot suggestions might provide, unless you intentionally plan to reduce your stress, it's never going to happen. Remember our discussions about goals? If you aim at nothing, you'll hit it every time. So get intentional about reducing your stress. None of us will develop a program of stress management unless we really plan to do so. Remember the story about the mother who came home and found her children playing with baby skunks? She had no plan for this emergency so she just yelled, "Run, children!!"

Each child grabbed a skunk and ran.

The following are several suggestions for stress reduction. Select a few that appeal to you and put them to work in your life.

1. Identify your stress. Become conscious of the stress in your life. There are various ways to do this. A questionnaire could help. Robert Eliot suggests that a stress test could consist of only one question: "In life, are you winning?" If you answer "No," chances are good that you're dealing with some stress in your life.

I'd recommend a longer version. There are various stress-awareness tests available. There is one at the end of this chapter that will give you a start in identifying your stress. Becoming aware of your stress may be as simple as recognizing how it affects you physically. A friend of mine breaks out in a rash. I feel stress in my shoulders. Others experience headaches. You need to become conscious of your own warning signal(s). These are the most common manifestations of stress (as researched by Priority Management Systems) and the percentage of people who reported them as stress indicators:

Headaches	33.1%
Anger	22.6%
Frustration	20.8%
Tension	7.9%
Fatigue/Tired	7.3%
Stomach Problems	5.9%

When your personal alarm goes off, you'll want to start implementing some of the stress relievers you're learning about in this chapter.

2. Breathe deeply. Become conscious of your breathing patterns and deliberately set aside times to take a few deep breaths every day. Everyone needs oxygen deep inside, but most people don't take enough time to breathe deeply.

You might want to start when you wake up in the morning. Sit up as straight as possible on the edge of your bed. Breathing in through your nose, take a deep breath all the way to the bottom of your lungs. Hold it while you slowly count to five (that can be increased to eight after a few days). Release the breath slowly through your mouth while counting silently to ten. Repeat that process five times before leaving the bed.

You can do the same while waiting at stoplights when driving, or at your desk at work. Make this a habit.

3. Meditate. Take some time for meditation or devotional thinking every day. Meditation literally means "to mull over." It is relaxing to spend some quiet time reflecting on thoughts that are calming for you. Many of us meditate by thinking about God, reading and thinking about sections of Scripture, or reading and reflecting on devotional materials. You may focus on something like the Serenity Prayer: "God, grant me the serenity to accept the things I cannot change, the courage to change the things I can, and the wisdom to know the difference." One variation on that prayer that I find meaningful is, "God, grant me the serenity to accept the people I cannot change, the courage to change the people I can change, and the wisdom to know that I am the only one I can change."

Find the material that helps you, and use it.

4. Relax. Develop your own relaxation sequence. It is often helpful to use a relaxation tape, made by someone else or by yourself. There is a script for progressive relaxation in appendix B. If you record yourself reading that script, you can then lie down or sit comfortably with your eyes closed and relax to the sound of your own voice talking you through the calming sequence.

Once you're feeling a level of deep relaxation, take a deep breath while thinking, "I am breathing in relaxation, peace, health, and energy." Then exhale and think, "I am breathing out all my tensions, fears, and frustrations." If you do this several times, your body develops a muscle memory and begins to identify the deep breath with deep relaxation. That makes your deep breathing doubly effective. The next time you feel stress coming on and can't get away to a quiet place, you can take a deep breath. Your body will remember!

5. Control time. Managing your time well is a great stress reducer, and you control the way you use your time. You set your own priorities. Take responsibility for using time to greater advantage. Make a checklist of the things you want to get done during the day, then list them in order of importance. Check off each item you accomplish. If you don't finish, carry the most urgent items over to the next day's list and begin again.

Set deadlines for yourself. I do this. If I have phone calls to make or to return, I list them and say to myself, "I will finish these by three this afternoon." Then I check them off as I make the calls.

Ken Blanchard's *One Minute Manager* is a helpful little book on time management that you might want to pick up and read. The key to managing time and stress is maintaining balance. The reason for this is that emphasizing one aspect of life over the others (which most people tend to do) generates stress. If others consistently accuse you of spending too much time doing something, listen to them! If you're working too many hours, deliberately schedule in play time and time for spiritual growth. You may need to do a time survey to determine where imbalances exist. This doesn't mean you spend the exact same amounts of time working, playing, exercising, meditating and resting. But you do want to make sure there's adequate time for each of these.

No one can tell you exactly how much time to devote to each activity in your life. Experiment, and make that determination for yourself. But getting control over your time and finding a good balance are important for controlling stress.

6. Network. Part of reducing your stress is developing a support system. Everybody needs somebody—including you. It's all right to let others help you.

One cancer patient shared with me how difficult it was for her to ask for help. Mary had always prided herself on being self-sufficient, and she valued being in control and being independent. Now she is learning not only to accept help, but even to ask for it. Now she has established a network of people who help her.

You may not even realize how competition has crept into the way you deal with others. It's a pervasive element in our society. But competitive attitudes get in the way of building support systems. Try to notice when you're feeling or acting competitive, and try to hold back. You don't have to lose all drive to help yourself heal, but you should stop trying to be stronger and better than everyone you meet. Such a competitive attitude drives others away, and it generates stress. It will be much easier to build a support system if you are not persistently competing with the people close to you.

Networking also means finding support among books and materials. Reading is another way we connect with those who have been through some of the same problems we have. It's stress-reducing to learn that others have overcome these problems. If you have some conscious problem areas, look for materials that will encourage you and help you find solutions.

7. Replace negatives with positives. You need to learn to say positive things to yourself. You can use the skills you are learning now to restructure your thought systems, replacing negatives with positives.

Start right here, with the stress reduction program you are developing. Begin saying positive things to yourself, such as, "I am learning to control the stress in my life. This will make me a healthier person." Repeat this ten times as you shower. Choose other positive statements to repeat at other spots in your daily routine.

One positive statement that has worked for me is thinking ahead to how I would handle being cut off in traffic. While driving in rush hour, I'd take a deep breath and say to myself, "I am not going to let inconsiderate people upset me today. I have decided this."

It's not wrong to give yourself positive affirmations. Remember the humorous beatitude, "Blessed are those who toot their own horns for, verily, they shall be well tooted." Applied in moderation, self-affirmation can be healthy. Try telling yourself: "I like myself. I enjoy people. I control my own stress. I have the courage to try. I am a survivor."

To eliminate some of the "negatives" in your life, stop complaining! It's true that life is often difficult and unfair. But you've got the right and ability to take what's around you and make the most of it—without complaining.

The alternative to complaining is finding solutions. Take the energy you would have wasted on complaining and turn it toward working on areas of difficulty.

In other words, "use the steam to move the engine, not just blow the whistle."

Dealing with the same problems over and over again is a consistent source of stress. For example, say you regularly show up late for appointments, excusing yourself because of the dreaded CLS (Chronic Lateness Syndrome). You can complain about the traffic problems, or receiving last-minute phone calls, or a broken zipper, or someone leaving your car with too little gas in the tank. But none of that complaining will get you anywhere on time. The solution? Stop complaining and start earlier. That will reduce stress.

Another way of letting go of negative emotions and experiences is to practice forgiveness. Grudges will make you sick and unattractive. Wasting energy on resentment is tragic; you need your energy for your health and wholeness.

I heard of two men who didn't speak to each other for more than ten years because they were angry over the placement of a fence that separated their properties. They were members of the same church and finally were confronted by a young pastor about the problem. Neither could remember the original source of the conflict. Still, for ten years, they'd wasted energy avoiding each other. Forgiveness is not only good for us spiritually, it is healthy.

Part of this new, positive thrust in your life could take the form of positive imaging. We don't know all the reasons this works, but it certainly seems to help. (Step Seven will give you more details on this subject.)

8. Watch your habits. To reduce stress, pay close attention to your habits. Now is the time to drop unhealthy ones, such as smoking (some think this is a relaxing habit; it actually stresses every blood vessel in your body) or drinking (drinking to relieve stress is a symptom of alcoholism).

Replace the bad habits you leave behind with healthy new habits, such as adequate sleep, exercise, and good nutrition. Few adults in America get enough sleep. We're a sleep-deprived nation! But adequate sleep will do wonders to reduce your stress.

Also, exercise releases the toxins caused by stress. Find some kind of appropriate physical exercise, and start to enjoy the benefits of exercise.

Author and exercise expert Dr. Kenneth Cooper told me that twenty to thirty minutes of aerobic exercise (exercise that increases the heart and breathing rates) every other day is sufficient for cardio-vascular conditioning and stress reduction. Personally, I do more than that, but my goal goes beyond stress reduction. I want to play basketball, so my routine includes running three miles five days a week and doing eighty sit-ups every other day. I sometimes add pull-ups or push-ups. Develop your own program and have your physician approve it according to current guidelines and his or her assessment of your needs.

Stress is also reduced by a nutritionally healthy diet. Find a balanced diet that works for you, then stick to it. I like a low-fat, low-sugar diet. I've included more fruits, too. I eat fruit early in the day and for snacking. Low-fat cereal is part of my breakfast menu (but I have to watch the labels to discover which cereals *really* are low in fats and high in fiber). Animal fat and most dairy products are no-nos for me. This diet has decreased my own stress level.

It pays to pay attention to the health advice of the experts. When, for example, they advise you to reduce the cholesterol in your diet, it's up to you to do it.

I can tell you, without fear of contradiction, the three most serious health problems in the world are: poorly managed stress (the causes vary, of course), dumb eating, and stupid habits. These are all things over which you and I have control. By exercising that control we will immediately improve our health and reduce our health costs.

9. Get outdoors more. We all spend too much time inside stress-producing environments. Even just living in close quarters every day generates stress for modern people. The closed-in feeling is often expressed in symptoms of stress.

So, spend some time outdoors. Take a walk in a park, drive out into the country and have a picnic at a roadside park, wade in a stream, sit and watch a sunset or sunrise, watch birds or squirrels play in the woods, or just lie down under the stars in your own back yard. Communing with nature can reduce your stress.

10. Be committed. Make a decision to feel better, and stick with your chosen program of stress reduction. No program is any better than the commitment to stick with it. Talking about programs of stress reduction can produce stress, but *doing* programs of stress reduction reduces stress.

Get motivated! Those who are most motivated to deal with their stress are those who have a sense of personal responsibility in dealing with their own health. They don't look around for someone or something else to blame for their problems. Their theme is "I am responsible." Accepting personal responsibility for your own stress reduction is healthy.

11. Celebrate life. The antithesis of stress is peace. Peace comes when we learn to celebrate and express gratitude for what we have.

Learn to celebrate your life. The following verses, called "The Iliad of the Day," may help you understand the meaning of celebration:

> I cross the threshold of the new day with reverence. It is my day to build or tear down. I choose to build it.
>
> This day will be filled, yet I will not haste it or waste it.
>
> My joy will be in serving and alleviating pain. My power will be in loving life.
>
> Arrogance I will not know. I will earn happiness by how I live.[1]

The way you celebrate will be unique to you. To me, celebrating life means being conscious for as much of the day as possible. I will be present in every conversation. I will focus on the events at hand. My mind will not drift from the tasks before me.

Wake up and live! To be alive is a celebration.

Just Do It

Obviously, health is improved by effective stress reduction. You can reduce your stress. Make sure you have a plan—a realistic plan. Stress management doesn't happen by itself; you have to make it happen. Your plan should include, at a minimum, these five elements:

- progressive muscle relaxation or a taped guide for muscle relaxation as described earlier
- regular deep breathing exercises
- exercise
- having fun
- variety

I also recommend reading a good book on stress reduction. Find one that works for you, then follow it! I recommend Robert S. Eliot's *Is It Worth Dying For?* or Robert K. Cooper's *Health & Fitness Excellence*.

What are you waiting for? Reducing stress in your life will bring the immediate benefit of feeling better every day and the long-range benefits of better health.

Participating This Week

The following questions may help you determine if you are presently stressed. Whether or not you have a high level of stress in your life, you will be healthier if you practice a good stress management program.

After looking over the questions, turn to the meditations for Step Four. Use them, and move one step closer to better health.

Step Four: Control Stress

Are You Stressed?

True (T) or False (F)
- ____ 1. The people with whom I work make me tense.
- ____ 2. When I am tense I relax by smoking or drinking.
- ____ 3. I frequently have pain in my neck and shoulders.
- ____ 4. I suffer from insomnia.
- ____ 5. I can't stop my thoughts at night.
- ____ 6. I have tension or migraine headaches.
- ____ 7. I often feel nervous or tense.
- ____ 8. I suffer from nervous indigestion.
- ____ 9. I have trouble concentrating because of worry.
- ____ 10. I take tranquilizers or sleeping pills to relax.
- ____ 11. It is hard for me to find time to relax.
- ____ 12. I live with constant deadlines. [2]

If six or more of these statements are true for you, you would be wise to follow up with further tests. One that I would suggest is the Life-Event test by Holmes and Rahe. This can be found in any public library. It is a test that measures accumulated stress resulting from various changes in life.

Stress is a major health problem. When unmanaged it results in retarding the immune system and causing us to become accident prone. Estimates of cost for stress-related illness have rocketed beyond $150 billion annually. It costs a lot more in human suffering. We will certainly be wise to develop the skill for managing stress in our daily lives. We will live longer and be healthier.

Notes

1. Walter Russell, as quoted in Glenn Clark, *The Man Who Tapped Secrets of the Universe* (n.p.: Macalaster Park, 1946).
2. Robert Eliot, *Is It Worth Dying For?* (New York: Bantam, 1989).

Chapter 7

Step Five: Develop Good Nutrition

I recently saw a man dumping salt on everything on his plate—vegetables, rice, and chicken. He kept shaking the salt on until he could see the little white grains clearly on his food. I asked him if he ever thought about cutting back on salt. He answered with a line that to me has become almost as bad as the salt: "My grandmother ate like this, and she lived to be 97."

I used to hear that same kind of rationalization in my own family. My family paid little attention to the fat, salt, cholesterol, or fiber content in our diets. I grew up in a home where fat was king. And here's how things came out.

My grandmother died at age 77 with arteries clogged in her legs. She literally died of gangrene due to poor circulation.

My grandfather didn't die until he was 80, but the last few years of his life were spent in a nursing home where he was totally out of touch with reality as a result of arteriosclerosis (hardening of the arteries). My uncle died of liver and pancreatic cancer about a year after surgery to replace the clogged arteries around his heart.

My father died of the effects of a stroke brought on in part by the eighty percent blockage in the arteries leading to his legs and partially as a result of his continued smoking. He used to be one of those people who laughed at the research and would say, "I get my exercise by serving as a pallbearer at the funerals of my friends who are health and exercise nuts." If that ever was funny, it isn't anymore.

Who can say whether they would have lived longer if they'd had different eating habits? I believe they would have. And I'm convinced that the quality of their lives would have been higher. I wish I could have made that fellow with the 97-year-old grandmother think twice about cutting back the salt content of his diet. Salt intake can exacerbate problems such as high blood pressure, heart muscle fatigue, kidney problems, and swelling (edema). I would have told him a second thing about his elderly grandmother. Our grandparents lived in a society with far less stress, and with cleaner water, air, and food. In such an environment, perhaps some folks could get away—at least temporarily—with less concern about nutrition and eating habits. But we don't live in that environment. We live in a high stress culture, and much of our environment is contaminated in one way or another. It's just common sense to balance our eating habits to offset a higher risk environment. Paying attention to and improving our diets is one way we add to our advantage.

Step Five: Develop Good Nutrition

Everybody's Talking about Fat

Have you noticed? Every time you turn around, someone is reporting new information about the dangers of fat in foods. The vast majority of nutritionists and health-care professionals today believe that fat constitutes the number-one health problem in America.

Nutritionist David Minz lists "The Ten Most Dangerous Food Problems." Here it is, from the least to the most dangerous:

10. *Pesticides.* These get into our diet on many of our fruits and vegetables and can mostly be avoided by buying organically grown produce. This is a serious problem, but it's not as high up the list as some expect it to be.
9. *Preservatives.* This is another problem but not as serious as we may have been lead to believe.
8. *Water.* It's not that the water is so bad; it's just that we don't drink nearly enough of it. Health experts estimate that we need six to ten glasses daily.
7. *Sugar and salt.* The average consumption of these two ingredients is astronomical in comparison to a person's need for them.
6. *Cholesterol.* We do not pay enough attention to the saturated fat content of our foods.
5. *Fat.*
4. *Fat.*
3. *Fat.*
2. *Fat.*
1. *Fat.*

Minz and others believe that fat in our diets is such a serious problem that it deserves all five of the top positions of the most dangerous food problems.

John A. McDougall, M.D., author of *The McDougall Plan* and *The McDougall Program* associates fat with disease of all kinds and recommends reducing fat content to between 10 and 15 percent of your calories per day.

I don't believe Dr. McDougall's opinion is extreme. If most people aimed at 10 percent they'd wind up eating about 20 percent of their calories in fat.

Do the Math (It's Easy)

Reducing your fat intake is not as difficult as it sounds. You can start by reading labels when purchasing packaged and canned foods. Legally, foods must be labeled. Check out the number of grams of fat in the food you are eating.

Here's how to figure the percentage of fat in a food: *Take the number of fat grams and multiply that by 9 (there are about 9 calories in each gram of fat). Divide the total number of calories for that food into the fat calories and you will have the percentage of fat in that item.* For example, if the label on your frozen dinner says that its total calories are 300 and that it contains 11 grams of fat. You can multiply the fat grams (11) by 9 (the number of calories in one gram). Eleven times nine equals ninety-nine. There are 99 fat calories in that food item. Next divide 300 (the total calories in the dinner) into 99 (the total fat calories in the dinner). The result of that division is 33.33. More than 33 percent of the dinner is fat. If you eat that, you will need to reduce your next meal to about 5 percent fat to balance it out.

For cleaner arteries, lower cholesterol, reduced risk of some cancers, and reduced risk of heart problems, keep your diet's fat content low! Aim at a maximum of 20 percent fat in total caloric intake.

This is NOT a diet. Unfortunately, the word "diet" is overworked—and misapplied. What most of us need is not a diet but a *permanent* change in eating style. And I emphasize the word *permanent*.

Making a permanent change in eating style won't happen with one bold step, but you can take small steps toward change. Maybe you could cut the fat content of breakfast for one month, then the next month concentrate on lunch. The goal would be to change and reduce the fat content of all your meals for the rest of your healthy life. Take a step, however small it may seem. For now, it's a step in the right direction.

What About Fiber?

Fat content is only one problem, though it is a major one. But it's wise to look at a few other areas of your diet as well.

Most of us don't get enough fiber in our daily fare. The result is constipation, colon problems, and hemorrhoids, for starters. There are other stomach problems associated with too little fiber.

Fiber for fat is a wise substitution. There is, however, a lot of misinformation about fiber. I have found that the richest fiber foods are kidney beans, brussels sprouts, cabbage, carrots, cauliflower, green beans, kale, peas, radishes, scallions, and tomatoes.

So what does fiber do that's so crucial for your health? Fiber absorbs water, thus increasing the size and softness of stool, and at least reducing the probability of hemorrhoids.

When it comes to fiber, the key is common sense. Eat the foods that grandma and mom used to ask you to eat. Eat vegetables and fruit—foods that are water-rich like apples, oranges, grapefruit, lettuce, carrots, greens, melons, grapes, bananas, etc. You will probably never eat too much fiber in natural foods.

Other Eating Problems

A few more common-sense changes can improve your nutritional level as well.

Vitamins. Vitamins as a supplement to your diet are usually a good idea, although you should talk with your doctor to determine the amount and which kind. Ask your doctor if he or she is familiar with nutrition. The fact that a person studied medicine is no guarantee that he or she has studied nutrition. Most doctors will refer you to someone else if necessary.

Choose what will be helpful to you. It certainly can help to get the advice of a professional nutritionist. Personally, I take a vitamin pack each day. This adds vitamins C, B complex, D, E, and some iron, protein, and beta-carotene to my intake.

Water. A minimum of sixty percent of your body is made up of water. Water forms the building blocks for cells and is the environment in which our cells live. Ninety-nine times out of a hundred, a person needs to raise his water intake.

Step Five: Develop Good Nutrition

Chew on this. In this hurried society people tend to hurry everything they do: We want fast food, instant oil changes, express banking, one-hour cleaning, short church services, and clear passing lanes on the freeway.

How many times have you eaten a meal that went like this: Get it fast, chew it three or four times, gulp down a drink and eat a candy bar on your way back to work? I'll admit, I used to do it. This is no exaggeration for many people I know. Does it sound familiar to you?

Don't hurry when it comes to chewing. Did you ever hear the long-lost rule, "Chew each bite twenty times before swallowing"? At least make it a goal to chew each bite ten times. It helps digestion.

Junk food. Most Americans eat far too much junk food—double cheeseburgers, quarter pounders, large fries, candy bars, chips, sodas, shakes and the like. We eat the excess fat calories, the excess cholesterol, the excess salt, and then one of us sues the restaurant franchise because they don't make the seats big enough for us to sit in.

Benjamin Disraeli said, "The health of the people is really the foundation upon which all their happiness and all their powers as a state depend." Do you want to be happy? Do you want to have more energy? Do you want to be healthier? In order to make a permanent change in your eating style, you've got to be totally committed to health. But this new lifestyle is a LIFEstyle—it can help you get well and stay well.

Eat less than twenty percent of your intake in fat. Drink at least six to eight glasses of water per day. Get plenty of fruit and vegetables.

Participating This Week

Check the appendix for meditations on nutrition and food intake. Think about better nutrition and practice it. Remember: No one cares more about your health and wholeness than you do. If you don't take charge of your eating habits, no one else can do it for you.

Chapter 8

Step Six:
Celebrate Life

Popular author Max Lucado tells a story that depicts a lot of lives. He says that Chippie the Parakeet never saw it coming. One second he was peacefully perched in his cage and the next he was sucked in, washed up, and blown over.

The problems began when Chippie's owner decided to clean Chippie's cage with a vacuum cleaner. She removed the attachment from the end of the hose and stuck it in the cage. The phone rang, and she turned to pick it up. She'd barely said "hello" when "sssopp!" Chippie got sucked in.

The bird owner gasped, put down the phone, turned off the vacuum, and opened the bag. There was Chippie—still alive, but stunned.

Since the bird was covered with dust and soot, she grabbed him and raced to the bathroom, turned on the faucet, and held Chippie under the running water. Then, realizing that Chippie was soaked and shivering, she did what any compassionate bird owner would do . . . she reached for the hair dryer and blasted the pet with hot air. Poor Chippie never knew what hit him.

A few days after the trauma, the reporter who'd initially written about the event contacted Chippie's owner to see how the bird was recovering. "Well," she replied, "Chippie doesn't sing much anymore—he just sits on his perch and stares."

Like Chippie's, songs have been stolen from a lot of hearts in this world. I see a lot of people who are just "sitting on their perches and staring." Many people have lost the joy of living; their energy for life is gone.

The sixth step toward health and wholeness is learning to enjoy life, which means, celebrate! Life, in spite of its hardships, can be a celebration. If we want to restore the song to our lives we must learn to celebrate in spite of it all. God did not put us on this earth just to "get by." We were created to enjoy God and the life we have been given. In enjoying life we honor the God who gave it to us.

Celebrate—Every Which Way You Can

We human beings celebrate all sorts of occasions. At the birth of a baby, we celebrate by taking pictures, sending and receiving cards, giving showers, and happily telling anyone who will listen about "the" baby. We celebrate graduations, anniversaries, and all kinds of accomplishments, victories and sales, holidays, seasons, and homecoming. We eat, dance, yell, laugh, sing, and tell. When celebration is not used as an occasion to abuse chemicals or corrupt our bodies, it is fun and healthy.

And you don't even need all these reasons. It has only been during the last few years that I've discovered that I don't need an excuse to have fun. I no longer wait for a special occasion. Celebration is so healthy that I plan or schedule it right into my life.

If you are a parent, celebrate with your children. For no reason other than your love for them, create a special moment for them. One person I know went to school and picked up her son at midday. She took him to a local planetarium, the place he chose for an outing. It was a special time that neither the mother nor the child will ever forget. She didn't wait for an occasion, she created one.

Create Special Moments

Frank decided to create a special moment for his ninety-year-old aunt on her birthday. She loves "Lara's Theme," so he hired an accordion player to come to her house and play that song for her. But he didn't just send the musician. He appeared at the door of her home with a card and gift and said, "Auntie, I know how much you love 'Lara's Theme' so I wanted to hire the New York Philharmonic Orchestra to come and play it for you today. But they couldn't make the trip, so this will have to do." With that the door opened and in walked the accordion player, playing the song for her.

She lived for a couple of years after that, and she often told Frank that he had given her the best birthday she had ever had. He had deliberately created a special moment for her. Do special things for the people you love. You don't have to have a reason. You make a reason.

Celebrating means doing nice things for you, too. Take yourself to a movie, buy yourself a gift, or go someplace that you have always wanted to visit. Build into your routine at least one special fun time for yourself each week.

Wake Up and Be Alive

Perhaps the true secret to enjoying life is simply staying awake—really living in the moment. I think multitudes of people doze right through life. Like Rip Van Winkle they sleep through revolutions.

Have you ever "slept" through anything? Have you ever driven several miles, then realized you hadn't even noticed where you'd been? Have you ever been in a conversation and suddenly realized you hadn't heard a word for the last five minutes? These things happen to everyone once in a while, but you can't let it become a lifestyle. It actually has become a lifestyle for some people.

Some people live in such a deep sleep that others just cannot reach them. Recently a woman was complaining about a man with whom she worked. She said, "He won't listen to me because I am a woman. He doesn't consider me important enough for him to care what I say."

She then smiled and mused aloud, "That shouldn't upset me, though, since he doesn't even listen to himself!"

Imagine—people so unaware that they not only do not listen to others, they don't even listen to themselves. Don't let it happen to you. WAKE UP! You really miss a lot by walking around like a zombie, sitting in front of a television set until you turn into a "couch-potato channel-changer" or drugging yourself into oblivion. You owe it to yourself to be conscious.

I hate missing *now*. My father used to say he hated to sleep at all. He said, "I would never sleep if I didn't just have to. You miss everything that's going on while you sleep."

Often when I am speaking in public, I begin by asking the audience to commit themselves to being "fully present" for my presentation. I know that the best use of time is to experience each moment as fully as I can, and I have more fun and enjoy my life more when I am awake.

Collect Funny Stories and Quips

You just never know when you're going to need a good laugh. So keep a collection of your own humorous books, funny stories, quips, and jokes.

Just to get you started, here's one from my collection:

> I am writing in response to your request for additional information. In block number 3 of the accident reporting form, I put "poor planning" as the cause of my accident. You said in your letter that I should explain more fully, and I trust that the following details will be sufficient:

I am a bricklayer by trade. On the day of the accident I was working on the roof of a new six-story building. When I completed my work, I discovered that I had about 500 pounds of bricks left over. Rather than carry the bricks down by hand I decided to lower them in a barrel by using a pulley, which fortunately was attached to the side of the building at the sixth floor.

Securing the rope at ground level, I went up to the roof, swung the barrel out and loaded the bricks into it. Then I went back to the ground and untied the rope, holding it tightly to insure a slow descent of the 500 pounds of bricks. You will note in block number eleven of the accident reporting form that I weigh 135 pounds.

Due to my surprise at being jerked off the ground so suddenly, I lost my presence of mind and forgot to let go of the rope. Needless to say, I proceeded at a rather rapid rate up the side of the building.

In the vicinity of the third floor, I met the barrel coming down. This explains the fractured skull and broken collarbone.

Slowed only slightly, I continued my rapid ascent, not stopping until the fingers of my right hand were two-knuckles deep into the pulley. Fortunately, by this time I had regained my presence of mind and was able to hold tightly to the rope in spite of my pain.

At approximately the same time, however, the barrel of bricks hit the ground—and the bottom fell out of the barrel. Devoid of the weight of bricks, the barrel now weighed approximately 50 pounds.

Step Six: Celebrate Life

I refer you again to my weight in block number eleven. As you might imagine, I began a rapid descent down the side of the building.

In the vicinity of the third floor, I met the barrel coming up. This accounts for the two fractured ankles and the lacerations on my legs and lower body.

The encounter with the barrel slowed me enough to lessen my injuries when I fell onto the pile of bricks and fortunately only three vertebrae were cracked.

I am sorry to report, however, that as I lay there on the bricks, in pain, unable to stand, and watching the empty barrel six stories above me, I again lost my presence of mind and I let go of the rope!

There's a story, and your collection is started. Now here are a few quips for your enjoyment.

Arrogance is bliss.
Abstinence makes the heart grow fonder.
Run it up the flag pole and see who sits on it.
Am I my brother's beeper?
No man can serve two masters with one stone.
Rome wasn't burned in a day.
It's on the fork of my tongue.
People who live in glass houses shouldn't throw sour grapes.

These came from a book you might want to read, *Splashes of Joy in the Cesspools of Life* by Barbara Johnson, a woman who has had many occasions for sadness or even despair in her life, but who chooses to celebrate. These laugh-lines were listed in a chapter titled, "Laugh and the World Laughs With You . . . Cry and You Simply Get Wet."

But why bother collecting stories and funny quips? Why look for ways to celebrate and have fun? Because having fun is healthy.

Having Fun Is Healthy

Josh Billings, a humorist quoted by Norman Cousins, said, "There ain't much fun in medicine, but there's a heck of a lot of medicine in fun." Such ideas are not being laughed at any longer. They are finding support in the established medical community. After Norman Cousins reported his personal experiences in *Anatomy of an Illness*, others have followed his lead in advocating the importance of having fun as a way of accelerating healing.

Cousins tickled himself by watching Marx brothers' movies and by watching the funniest episodes he could find from "Candid Camera." You can do the same thing. Find a type of movie or book or joke that makes you laugh, and treat yourself to it!

The *Journal of The American Medical Association* (27 January 1989) ran a report of a Swedish study on the effect of laughter on quality of life and symptom relief. It was titled "Laugh if This Is a Joke." The article reported that a humor therapy program can improve the quality of life for patients, and "laughter has an immediate symptom-relieving effect for these patients."

While emphasizing the value of laughter, Cousins reminds us that he uses laughter as a metaphor for the full range of positive emotions. While it may be hard for some people to understand how seriously ill patients can laugh or find humor in their situations, it is imperative for them to do so. And it is possible. The human mind is able to twist words, jump to illogical conclusions, and laugh in the most unlikely and paradoxical situations. An example of how creative the human mind can be in creating humor can be seen in W. C. Fields. He was able to see humor in selfish stinginess. He said he knew a man who was so stingy that he only allowed his son to have one measle at a time.

I visited my father after he had a serious surgery. He told me he wanted to go home from the hospital. I told him that he was where he needed to be to recover. He grinned, "Why, Bill, this is a terrible place for a person to get well. Just about everyone in here is sick. I might catch something."

He found a way to laugh even in painful situations. When he had a stroke in 1992, we took him to the emergency room at a local hospital. The examining physician wanted to check the extent of the damage to his face so he asked, "Can you smile, Mr. Little?"

My dad responded, "If I had something to smile about I could." He never lost his sense of humor. It helped him recover from some very serious illnesses and made even the painful times easier.

No wonder Voltaire said, "The art of medicine consists of amusing the patient while nature cures the disease."

Laughter as Painkiller

Most of us have become familiar with the pioneering work by Norman Cousins. He really made us conscious of the power of humor. His oft-quoted observation is still revolutionary: "I learned that ten minutes of genuine belly laughter had an anesthetic effect and would give me at least two hours of pain-free sleep."

Having a good belly laugh won't affect all of us in the same way, but it will relieve pain to some degree in any of us. The biblical writer of the book of Proverbs understood this when he wrote, "A cheerful heart is good medicine" (17:22).

Humor as Stress Relief

A woman who calls herself "A. Pixie" was recently in my office talking about how her family seemed to have deserted her. Ms. Pixie was philosophical about it, though, and said that her friends had become her family. She eased her own pain with, "They say that blood is thicker than water, but you can live a lot longer on water than on blood, unless you are a vampire."

Her sense of humor was delightful. Would you believe this is the same lonely lady who had once told me she'd stopped answering her phone because it was always just a wrong number? She'd learned to let humor carry her through her difficulties.

My dad said, "If you have personality and a sense of humor, you don't have anything to worry about." There's no doubt about it, humor reduces stress and worry. To live without humor makes about as much sense as setting your hair on fire and then using a hammer to put it out.

Humor Is Where You Find It

Comedian Mel Brooks says, "Life literally abounds in comedy if you just look around you. We can find humor in a hospital room, an office, in church. It is a matter of mindset. Look for a laugh and you'll find it."

In one church on Easter Sunday, the minister announced that during the "next hymn, Mrs. Johnson will come to the front and lay an egg on the altar."

A child in my church's Vacation Bible School was looking for a gray crayon. When his teacher asked him why, he replied that he wanted to color God. The teacher asked, "How do you know to color God gray?"

The boy answered, "Because when we pray before we eat, we say 'God is gray, God is good. Let us thank him for our food.'"

I once asked a parishioner if she heard a statement I had made in my sermon. I still wonder if it was a slip of the tongue when she answered, "No, I don't hear everything you say from the 'bullpit.'"

Life is awfully funny. There's humor everywhere. Learn to watch for it. Take time to laugh. It makes you well and keeps you healthy.

Participating This Week

Be sure to look at the seven meditations on this topic. I hope they help you remember to laugh, because laughter is not only the music of the soul, it is healing for the body.

Chapter 9

Step Seven: Envision Wholeness

I once read a story about a young prince who had a crooked back. This caused him to stand in a twisted position. The king commissioned a sculptor to make a statue of his son. In his imagination, the sculptor delivered the crippled prince from his deformity. He gave the statue regal bearing and a handsome, healthy appearance. The statue looked exactly like the prince but without deformity.

Every day for months the prince sat in the garden, gazing at the image of what he might have been. He dreamed of looking so straight and tall. So gradually that he hardly noticed, he stood more and more erect, until one day he looked into a mirror, and there was looking back at him the image of a man standing straight and tall. As he had constantly gazed at the statue, he had become like it.

This fairy tale holds an element of truth. We do become our visions of ourselves. What we see is not only what we get, but also what we become. The dreams and images that we hold consistently in our mind's eye drastically influence our future selves. In his book, *Greatest Discovery,* Earl Nightingale calls visualization "a force of incalculable power."

Visualization is the mind's picture of our expectations—and people grow into their expectations. Theodosius Dobzhansky wrote, "Tell me what your vision of the future is, and I will tell you what you are."

What do you envision? Like the prince, you need healthy models. What pictures fill your imagination? Are they images of heart attacks, cancer, accidents, losing, failing, being fired, being cheated on or lied to? How many nights have you drifted off to sleep worrying about problematic scenarios that *might* take place?

If you want to be healthy, you will be helped if you stop negative thinking. Leaving behind the negative images begins with deciding to focus on positive images.

Unhealthy Role Models

While in seminary, I was contemplating a study on demons and demon activity. But one of my professors warned me against this, saying, "You become what you study." He feared that I would spend too much time on the subject of evil. He wanted me to be careful.

Many people study too many "demons." Medical research focuses time and money to study the sick and too little time researching healthy role models. All the media know that people are more interested in the sick or sensational than the wise and healthy. When was the last time you picked up a magazine or book and read "How I Never Became Sick" or "The Emotional

Profile of a Person Who Has Never Been Depressed and Never Even Thought of Suicide"?

In high school assemblies, they bring in young people who have "kicked" the drug habit. I'm glad for these young people, and they deserve congratulations. But why not honor young people who never developed the habit? Wouldn't they make better role models?

When I set out fifteen years ago to do a study on healthy marriages, I found very little literature on that topic. Nobody at that time was writing about couples who have never had marital conflict. No, all the literature focused on marital problems and failures. (Fortunately, that situation has been rectified in recent years, especially in the Christian publishing world.)

Our books and magazines tend to describe drug abuse, sexual perversions, suicide, and mental and physical illness. No wonder suicide rates are up, deviant behavior is rampant, and hospitals are filled with physically and mentally ill people. We should be studying people who are models of physical and mental health. Our students need role models who are successful and have never used drugs. I want to see some movies about honest, healthy people living according to basic values.

But change isn't imminent, and it's no one's fault but our own. No one would pay to see the movie about healthy people. Even popular children's movies focus on things like murderous sibling rivalry *(The Lion King),* wicked stepmothers *(Snow White),* desires to be something one is not *(The Little Mermaid),* and other unhealthy human and animal dynamics. We'll continue to see a flood of material on sick society because that's what we buy. That is a frightening prospect, because we do indeed become what we see modeled.

We have never needed healthy role models more than we do today. We desperately need mentors and models among the healthy and the survivors. I recently read about a thirty-nine-year-old man who had established a highly successful business as a stock broker. The stock market crash of October, 1987, however, left him bankrupt. In the midst of business failure, his mental problems escalated. His wife left him. In the end, he pointed a .38 revolver at his temple and pulled the trigger. He had no coping skills, no models for successfully dealing with life's hardest blows.

The Healthy Person's Character

We all need those models. Over the last fifteen years, I have studied numerous patients who recovered from serious illness, and I have looked at the lives of healthy people who have stood the test of years. I have talked to friends and family members, and from all their observations has come what I call the "Healthy Model." These survivors and healthy people have some characteristics in common.

Balance. First, healthy people maintain balance. They are not Johnny One Notes who have only one focus. Their interests are varied. They enjoy time alone and still maintain a social life. They blend work and play. Free to express their independence, healthy people are also free to accept help from others.

My dad was an excellent example of the kind of healthy person I am describing. I call him a poor man's philosopher because he never wrote a book nor attained much formal education. In fact, he attended school for fewer than eight years. It wasn't that he didn't want an education; he just came along at a time when he couldn't continue in school. Still, he never let that stop him from expressing sweeping ideas about life.

"I have opinions on prackly everything," he would say. "And I's usually right. At least I think I am, but I guess everyone else thinks he is too."

Dad not only never took himself too seriously, but he helped me not to take myself too seriously. When I talked with him about writing this book, he said, "Keep it simple, make it entertaining, and don't try to say too much. Most people are like me [one of his basic assumptions], and we want easy entertainment when we read. We don't want to learn a lot. I already know all I want to know. I just read for fun."

But he makes a great point: People probably learn more when they are entertained.

Psychologist Rollo May said, "Freedom is the ability to pause between a stimulus and a response and in that pause make a decision about what we want to do." Balance means thinking and exercising our freedom to choose our reactions in moments of relaxed attention. It means not permitting a failure to become devastating. It means taking time to play and enjoy the world around us. It means daring to go barefoot once in a while. Balance your life.

Sense of humor. Second, healthy people do not take themselves too seriously. Life is just too important to be taken seriously. People who are wearing constant frowns are usually not living healthy lives. Healthy role models view themselves in a lighthearted way. But unhealthy people take themselves too seriously, and they get upset when others do not take them just as seriously.

Healthy people have a lot of fun. So many people value laughter as a healing force that laugh clinics have sprung up all across the country to teach people how to laugh. Isn't that a commentary? Now we have to be taught how to laugh. Laughter is so natural that all we have to do is listen to a bunch of children playing to hear it. It is a shame that we forget how to have fun.

My philosophical dad even turned work into fun. "I really have fun at work," he used to say. "I have to spend eight hours a day there, so I am going to have fun." He knew that he could enjoy work because his worth and value were not in his job but in himself.

Having fun is healthy. Laugh a lot, even if you have to watch old slapstick movies as Norman Cousins did. Find funny jokes and fun activities. If you have a friend you can laugh with, cultivate that friendship. Spend time with that friend and stay away from the Gloomy Gusses. When you look at healthy people you will see them balancing work and play.

No worry. Third, healthy people do not worry much, if at all. I once asked my dad how he handled worry. After his characteristic deep breath and raised eyebrows, he said, "Worry is a word that should be taken out of the dictionary. As long as it's in there, people will think they are supposed to do it. The only reason I can figure for anyone to worry is that he must think he

"How about money as a cause of worry?" I persisted.

"Why, Bill," Dad mocked, "if you have money, you don't need to worry. If you don't have money, you shouldn't waste time worrying about it. You should go out and try to earn some.

"There just aren't many reasons to worry. Dying?" Dad asked the question of himself. "You have known you were going to die since you were this high." He held his hand, palm down, about two feet above the floor. "Since you know it's going to happen, and you can't do anything about it, you might as well go ahead and live while you can.

"Worrying just never made any sense to me," my dad went on. "It never earned a penny, never saved a life, never made anyone well. Right now, I'm worried about being thirsty. Hand me a soda."

I obliged Dad with a soda, and he took a drink and smiled at me. "Now I'm not worried about that anymore."

My father's attitude is a practical application of the Serenity Prayer: "God grant me the serenity to accept the things I cannot change, courage to change the things I can, and the wisdom to know the difference."

I heard a successful cancer doctor say that the best way to health is to "choose peace, and leave your troubles to God." Worry is useless, but it is worse than that. Worry never solves anything—and it can make you sick. Jesus told us, "Do not worry about your life, what you will eat or drink; or about your body, what you will wear." We are to take as our example the birds. "They do not sow or reap or store away in barns, and yet your heavenly Father feeds them. Are you not much more valuable than they? Who of you by worrying can add a single hour to his life?" (Matthew 6:25-27). Of course, this sometimes takes more faith than we have. But read over the whole of Matthew chapter 6 and savor the sense that God will take care of you if only you will let him.

Hope. Fourth, healthy people are hopeful. Another sign of my dad's good health was his hopefulness in situations that would make most people turn and run. Healthy people believe there is always a way out, a solution to every problem, a cure for every sickness. When they appear to be trapped, they look for answers, not excuses, and they never give in to despair.

Once Dad and I were riding on a two-lane street in Chicago with my brother, Larry. Rain was falling, and traffic was at a standstill. The left lane seemed to be open, so Dad suggested that Larry pull out in it to pass the traffic.

"We might meet other cars," Larry protested.

"Naw," said Dad. "Pull on around this truck. You've got plenty of time." He always sounded convincing.

Larry drove out into the left lane. Bad decision. Traffic was meeting us head on!

Dad spoke hurriedly with a smile in his voice. "Throw it in reverse."

Larry had decided by now to go ahead and hope the truck would permit him back in the right lane. "What good will it do to throw it in reverse?" It was more of a statement of irritation than a question.

"Well, when they hit you, you can say you were backing up." My dad grinned, as if to say he could always find a way out.

People who feel blocked in will give up in despair. People who believe there is a way out will grin and "throw it in reverse." Look for solutions. Look for the bright side. It's good for your health.

Responsibility. Fifth, healthy people take responsibility for themselves. As we used to say in southeast Missouri, "Every tub has to sit on its own bottom."

This is not such an easy thing to do. Once at a family reunion, my dad took a terrible ribbing because, a few years earlier, he had driven more than halfway from St. Louis to Mississippi and turned around because it was too far to drive at one time. Later I asked him why he had done that. He said, "I don't think I did."

"Then why didn't you just tell them that you hadn't done it?"

He thoughtfully replied, "I couldn't do that. Last year I might have told them I did it."

If you tell tall tales, you have to pay the consequences. We have to pay the consequences for a lot of things in life. Healthy people do so because they accept responsibility for themselves.

I was recently asked what one thing I would say is the single most important advice anyone could give. I responded by saying that the most important thing anyone can know is that each person is responsible for himself or herself. Everyone has a choice about how he or she will respond to life's situations.

If you take responsibility, you will participate in your own health care. You'll stop smoking, reduce alcohol intake, cut back on salt, reduce animal fat, maintain healthy weight levels, eat more fruit and vegetables for fiber, take vitamins and minerals, plan stress reduction, exercise regularly, have fun, set goals, establish personal faith, and maintain balance. Chances are you've already done several of these.

People who take responsibility do not wallow in guilt or self-pity. They do not blame others, their race, sex, financial status, or anything else for their own shortcomings. Responsible people take whatever situation they face and make the most of it without complaining.

It seems clear to me that those of us who are willing to take responsibility for our own lives have a chance to be much healthier than people who view themselves as victims. Victims simply look for ways to suffer. They are more likely to use an illness or problem as an excuse than to look for ways to improve themselves.

Taking responsibility means that when we are confronted with a problem we will put forth effort to solve it. I have never known a healthy person who just sat on his "backside." My dad's attitude toward solving problems was, "Somebody messed this world up before I got here, so I have to do what I can to straighten it out."

Take responsibility for yourself.

The Power of Imagery

One way we can take responsibility for ourselves and our healing is by using imagery. The power of visual images has been well documented. The benefits have been especially dramatic in healing, selling, and in the performance of athletes. One major-league pitcher, Matt Young, was at a dead end in his career. Matt could not control his pitches. Then he started using relaxation with imagery. Three times a day, he relaxed and listened to an audio tape I made for him. The tape described an exercise in imagery in which he would see himself on the mound from the time he got the signal from the catcher for a specific pitch, through his windup and delivery. He was instructed to see himself in perfect form and balance and then to see the ball arriving in the strike zone, right where he wanted it. He was told to see himself as if he were watching himself on television.

Matt was to see the process, feel the balance, and hear the response of his teammates congratulating him on the good pitches he made. In other words, he played the game in his mind. The result was that he consistently pitched better when he faithfully listened to his tapes.

In several newspaper interviews, Matt credited this exercise with saving his career and making him an All-Star pitcher representing the Seattle Mariners. "Without this help," he said, "I'd be hanging wallpaper instead of pitching for a salary of six figures a year."

I have worked with pitchers, hitters, football players, basketball players, weight lifters, swimmers, divers, golfers, and tennis players. All have benefited from using visual rehearsal. The improvement of their performances was easy to measure and easy for observers to note. Improvement in performance followed envisioning improvement in performance.

Step Seven: Envision Wholeness

This type of exercise has also been beneficial in sales training. One major company with which I have been privileged to work has used my tapes to help in sales performance. I made a relaxation and imagery tape for their sales training department. They use it for all new salespeople and as a review for experienced sales people.

We begin with relaxation because it is easier to picture and retain what we see if we are relaxed. The sales tape talks the salespeople through a sales call. They are instructed to see themselves responding quickly and confidently to questions from potential customers. They see themselves following through on each step of the sale.

Salespeople report that the tape and the process help them feel more comfortable, remember their goals, and perform at higher levels than before using the tape.

The key in using such imagery is to see things happening the way you want them to happen and to use the tape or envisioning exercise at least two to three times per day.

Of course, visualization has helped many patients in their battle against cancer. The use of imagery or visualization with cancer patients was popularized by Carl and Stephanie Simonton, whose work is described in their book *Getting Well Again*. While I do not agree with their entire perspective, they have much of value to say.

I ask cancer patients to use imagery for three reasons. First, when you form clear visual images of a potential reality, you increase the likelihood of its becoming a reality. It acts like a self-fulfilling prophecy.

An image becomes a vision or a pictorial goal and acts like a magnet, moving you toward it. If you imagine yourself healthy and picture health in your mind, you increase your chances of achieving health.

Many cancer patients use this process to help restore health to their bodies. They picture their white blood cells, the workers in the immune system, fighting cancer. Each person uses his or her unique pictures. Some see their white cells as piranha fish attacking and destroying the cancer cells in their bodies. Others see the immune system functioning like PacMan™ in a video game. Some see armies of medical people in their blood, working for healing. Others picture God sending out power for recovery. Research (most notably by Jean Acterberg) shows that people who practice seeing these images three or more times every day seem to fight cancer consistently better than those patients who do not participate in their healing programs through imagination.

To envision can also be to imagine we see images, even if at first we cannot. Some people close their eyes and immediately see clear pictures. Others close their eyes and see nothing but darkness. A patient's wife recently called me and said that the patient had become discouraged about this process because he couldn't see anything when he closed his eyes. I urged him to use the process anyway. We are better at imagining than we realize, and we can improve with practice.

The second reason I recommend using imagination is that, if you cannot imagine a thing, then you may have trouble believing it. And without being able to believe it, you have no hope. Hope provides energy for action and health. If you could not imagine Christ living on earth, traveling around the Jordan, and dying on a cross, might you have difficulty believing it? Thinking in pictures about Christ's birth, life, death and resurrection is the same as envisioning it. You are creating a mental picture of Christ. Where would we be without those mental pictures?

In a sense, then, "seeing" is believing and believing is "seeing." Beliefs shape our emotions, reactions, and behaviors. The visualization process is simple and powerful. Decide what you want to achieve and then practice seeing it a least three times a day. What a difference it would make to our lives if we frequently envisioned Christ walking beside us day by day. We believe it, but how much more powerful it is when we have a mental picture of it!

The third reason I recommend using mental imagery is that it gives the patient something to do. One of the devastating things about cancer is that it places us out of control. We feel better when there is something that we can do for ourselves. This gives us something concrete that we can do.

It Works if You Work It

Many start, few finish. Some folks make short-term gains with the use of visualization. Then they quit. They become bored or tired or lose their motivation. The baseball pitcher to whom I referred earlier used his tape everyday for several weeks. Matt improved his performance and quit the process. His performance suffered immediately. He had to start over. I told him to "dance with the one that brought him to the dance." When it begins to work, keep working at it.

I'll admit that this kind of use of imagination is a little mysterious. No one seems to understand clearly why or how it works, though the evidence is clear that it does work. In Philippians 4:8 Paul instructs his listeners to "think about" (might that include picturing?) "whatever is true," "noble," "right," "pure," "lovely," "admirable," "excellent," and "praiseworthy." Imagine the power of filling our minds with such things!

But the fact that we don't understand how it works is practically irrelevant. When Sir Alexander Fleming found that a little mold spore had landed in his experiment and killed off bacteria in a circle around the spore, he didn't understand the mechanism, but he knew that penicillin might be a powerful agent in fighting disease.

Don't wait to use imagery until we understand why imagery works. Use it now. Become what you envision.

Participating This Week

By now you've established a good pattern of using the daily meditations that will encourage you toward health. Look for the meditations in the appendix and let them help you get started in seeing and believing.

Chapter 10

Step Eight: Exercise Healthy Spirituality

When a colleague and I started plans to establish a cancer/health support center in St. Louis, we contacted a group that had experience and a national reputation with such projects. After discussing their program at length we were brought to an abrupt halt by one statement. We were told, "If you start a center using our name, there can be no spiritual focus. Spiritual matters are off limits for us."

How could we work to support cancer patients and promote good health without a spiritual focus anywhere in the program? We could not!

Frequently the first questions I am asked by cancer patients relate to faith in God, prayer, and what will happen after death. To ignore this would be to fail to support the patients and to fail in education for health.

Andy was a patient with glioblastoma (a form of cancer of the brain). The first contact I had with him was in a hospital room. I'd joined him to talk about stress reduction.

"How can I help you?" I asked.

With tears in his eyes and a tremor in his voice he pleaded, "Please teach me how to pray."

We started with the basics of belief. He learned to pray the child's prayer:

> Now I lay me down to sleep,
> I pray the Lord my soul to keep.
> If I should die before I wake,
> I pray the Lord my soul to take.

He was comforted by that prayer, and we were then ready to deal with other critical issues related to the illness.

Mary was near death because of small cell carcinoma of the lungs. She was teary-eyed as we talked in her hospital room.

"What gives you the strength to keep fighting?" I asked with honest admiration.

She responded with a smile, "You may think this is silly, but when I am afraid I sing, 'Jesus loves me, this I know, for the Bible tells me so . . .'"

I didn't think that was silly at all.

Healthy Religion Increases Physical Health

I focus on spiritual issues, not only because people ask these questions and gain strength from their faith, but because I believe that healthy spirituality is physically healthy.

Step Eight: Exercise Healthy Spirituality

Are religious people healthier than non-religious people? The answer is probably yes. Certainly there are forms of religion that hinder, rather than help, but healthy spirituality is surely healthy. Unhealthy, rigid, judgmental, negative, guilt-producing religion is unhealthy.

But generally, people of faith *are* healthier than people without faith. The following are excerpts from a poll taken by *Christianity Today* (23 November 1992):

> Men who went to church and liked it had much lower BP's [blood pressures] than men who didn't go to church and didn't care about religion....
>
> Church attendance, prayer, and the social support available at church were frequently found to be significant positive factors in helping patients with mental or physical health problems....
>
> Religious commitment lowers rates of mental disorders, drug use, and school drop-out....
>
> Religious people who live out their faith are more likely to say they are enjoying life, that they like their work, their marriage, their family.

The operative phrases from these excerpts are "went to church and liked it" and "live out their faith." Simply being a member of a religious group or a church is no guarantee that one has a healthy spirituality. That faith, that spirituality has to give to a person's life a sense of meaning, a reason to live in healthy ways, a sense of personal worth, a community of interpersonal support, and a hope for the future both before and after death. I have found that Christianity offers that to those who are seeking. But even the Christian religion can be unhealthy when it closes minds to the helpful truths of medicine, science, psychology, and human relations. It is possible to embrace Christianity outwardly and still be as empty as a hole in the ground spiritually. When spirituality leads to love and acceptance of others as well as a commitment to alleviate human suffering, it is healthy.

There is certainly a connection between religion and health. That connection, unfortunately, can be damaging as well as beneficial. That occurs especially when legalistic religion promotes the negatives of extreme guilt, rejection, and fear, when the religion keeps an individual from seeking proven and available treatments for illness, and when it identifies sickness with sin. People who have serious illness certainly do not need inappropriate guilt heaped on them.

The relationship between religion and health is positive when religion focuses on acceptance, love, forgiveness, peace, and grace. These are the characteristics of religion as presented by Jesus Christ in the Bible.

I assert that healthy spirituality not only makes people healthier, it also helps physically sick people get well.

The Spiritual Issue

Spirituality may be defined as the belief that there is something more than this material existence, that there is meaning beyond this world, that there is Someone or something greater than the visible world, that somewhere exists a creative force, a reality beyond finite life. For me and many others, that power is a personal God; that power rests in Jesus Christ. I deal with this issue because when people are facing life-threatening illness they have a tremendous concern for meaning and for questions about death and beyond.

The importance of this issue is brought home to me again and again in my office. John, a cancer patient, sat in my office holding his wife's hand as he said, "The best thing that has happened out of this terrible disease is that I am beginning to understand the meaning and purpose of my life."

Another reason for emphasizing healthy spirituality is that sick people are often overwhelmed with guilt. They believe that God is punishing them for some reason, or that they are supposed to get some message from this illness. There are times when disease is directly related to one's behavior, such as smoking, but there are even more times when it is not. We all suffer from the damage done to our environment, our water supply, and to our foods. We suffer from passive smoke. We are affected by other things over which we have no control. We live in a fallen world where destructive forces have an impact. We know that it rains on both the just and the unjust, but sometimes it rains even more on the just because the unjust steals the just's umbrella.

These are spiritual issues *and* health issues. We need to address them specifically.

Healthy Spirituality

Health in spiritual matters begins with having the courage to believe in something beyond ourselves. In describing survivors of cancer, Bernie Siegel says that they have faith in their doctors, faith in themselves, faith in medicine, and faith in God. Faith, the substance of things hoped for and not seen, is an essential ingredient in a spirituality that contributes to physical health.

The need for positive faith in medicine is well documented by myriad studies on the power of placebos. People get sick when they believe a "pill" will make them sick, and they often get better when they believe a "pill" will make them better. In both cases they have been given a sugar pill; the effect was not the result of the pill but beliefs about it. Certainly faith in a medication will enhance the effect of that medication.

The kind of faith we have is also important. It is not enough just to believe; we must believe in something. We may believe in God, but fail to see that the kind of God we believe in will influence our direction. An active faith in a God of love who wants us to be physically better and wants to free us of pain is certainly more conducive to health than a faith in a vindictive God who arbitrarily sends illness on us or punishes us with illness. Positive faith that results in action toward health is a tremendous asset in the healing process and in wellness in general.

Healthy spirituality involves prayer and meditation. Bill Moyers is among several Americans to begin to develop an interest in the powerful mental approaches of the Chinese and other eastern philosophies and religions. His work on *Healing and the Mind* gives a new legitimacy to the connection between prayer, meditation, and physical health. Moyers has made us aware of some Eastern techniques for meditation.

In the Christian tradition, meditation has an added dimension. We are not only to clean and empty our hearts of evil and unhealthy spirits but to fill them with good. (Note Matthew 12:43-45.) It is not enough to stop thinking negative thoughts. We need to replace them with positive ones. It is not enough to empty our minds. We must fill them with thoughts that are healthy. One way to achieve this is by focusing attention on our favorite Psalm. We may also focus on truth, honesty, justice, purity, loveliness, goodness, and virtue (Philippians 4:8). Meditate on these things. They are lovely.

I believe that reflective meditation or quiet times of prayer can enhance our health. It is essential to maintaining balance. The hurried pace of life has to be slowed down to give us time to examine ourselves. It takes a strong philosophy or deep sense of spirituality to cope with the demands of life, and that cannot be developed without quiet reflection and time for decision-making. Meditation, relaxation, and prayer contribute to health.

Healthy spirituality gives unity to attitudes and behaviors. It fits seamlessly into our lives. It is not phony pietism or pretended strength. It is real. When your spirituality fits with your life, it is believable. That fit makes what you say sound real. If you don't really believe what you say you believe, it will be readily apparent. You don't need to pretend to be something you are not. You don't have to wear plastic smiles when you are actually in pain.

This true-to-life faith is a major point in the biblical book of James, which says that faith and works (deeds) must go together. Integrity in faith means that you are not pretending to believe things that others think you should believe. Living a lie dissipates energy and can make you sick. Honest faith contributes to your healing and health. Jesus said, "You will know the truth, and the truth will set you free" (John 8:32). When you live in a manner that matches your faith, you are free.

Healthy spirituality is balanced. Balance, another key concept in producing a healthy life, is also included in a healthy spiritual life. Let's consider several kinds of balance that grow out of a healthy spiritual base and see how they relate to good health.

First, there is balance between tolerance of others and freedom to express your own ideas and faith. Whether you have a religious faith or not, you have the right to express your views. I suffered for many years because I was reluctant or embarrassed to express my personal faith. I was tolerant of others, and I still am. But now I expect to be tolerated, too.

I have become bolder in my personal expression and more honest in my tolerance in the passing of the years. There is boldness in healthy spirituality. That is part of the freedom to be yourself. In your everyday life, you don't have to be afraid to say out loud what you are, what you feel, and what you believe. When you discover how important it is to express yourself, you will begin to work on the courage to do it.

I remember once riding on the bow of a fishing boat on the Gulf of Mexico. I was enjoying the beautiful sight of the rolling waves—until a queasy feeling came over me. "It's just in my mind," I thought, "and besides, if I do get sick, I'll stay right here and never tell my family and that group gathered at the stern of the boat."

My pride lasted for about three minutes. Soon I was staggering through the crowd of about thirty people, green-faced. I had lost all concern about admitting that I was sick. I think I was shouting, "I'm sick." I walked through the crowd and into the captain's cabin.

The captain said, "Hey, you can't go in there."

I didn't even respond. I just went on in and laid down on his bunk. There comes a time when you know you must express yourself. You don't, however, have to wait until you're sick to do it!

The closer I come to the culmination of life, the less concern I have about appearing to be intellectual or popular. I just want to be real. So I wander through the crowds on the stern of the boat of life saying, "I have faith in God. I believe in Jesus Christ." Healthy spirituality is always characterized by a balance of boldness and tolerance.

Second, healthy spirituality is a faith that includes balance between conviction and flexibility. Personal faith necessitates strong conviction. While I want to remain flexible enough to learn from others, I also acknowledge that I have gambled everything on my faith that Jesus is the Christ. It has been said that if we don't stand for something we will fall for anything.

We must have the courage to live according to our own values. Failure to do so will create inner turmoil and stress, and we have already seen how devastating stress can be.

On the other hand, you must retain enough humility to acknowledge that, even in your wisdom, you do not know everything. Humility necessitates flexibility. On a practical level, it also makes sense to be flexible. The more flexible you are, the more resources you have. Healthy and successful people maintain alternatives. If you block them, they find alternate routes to their goals or find new goals. Whether in religion or work, rigid, one-dimensional people are limited in their responses to life situations. When such people lose an arm, a leg, a breast, a spouse, or a job, they have fewer options. Their lives are more easily thwarted. Flexible people find another area of strength, another direction.

The story of W. Mitchell is well documented in numerous articles. Mitchell was indescribably burned in a terrible motorcycle accident. His injuries would have destroyed an inflexible person. Such a person would have whined, "Now I can't do what I wanted to do. My life is ruined." Thwarted in the direction he had expected his life to take, W. Mitchell simply changed his direction. He became a highly successful manufacturer of wood-burning stoves.

As if the burns were not enough, a second accident—this time in an airplane, left W. Mitchell paralyzed. But even this disability didn't stop him. He turned his energies toward politics.

One of my favorite quotes from Mitchell is, "Before all this happened to me there were probably 10,000

Step Eight: Exercise Healthy Spirituality

things I could have done. Now there are probably only 1,000. I am not going to focus on the 9,000 things that I can't do; I am going to focus on the 1,000 that I can do." What an inspiration!

Flexible people are survivors, so balance conviction and flexibility.

Third, you need the balance between resignation and the determination to make things better. Acceptance must be paired with commitment to change. Resignation that accepts things the way they are can make you an apathetic victim unless you balance it with a recognition that you are responsible for making life better wherever you can. You cannot see from God's vantage point, so you have to maintain enough humility to be willing to change.

One patient I saw recently said he had opted to continue chemotherapy after reading a book on fighting cancer. Initially he had simply hoped that God would heal him supernaturally. Now, he wants to trust God, but he also wants to do the best he can to use what God has provided for him through medical resources.

Some people identify their conditions with the will of God, deciding nothing they could do would improve their situation, because "God's will be done." Such an attitude blinds them to the help available.

I remember the frustration of working with Joan, a woman who had ovarian cancer. I encouraged her to use relaxation and imaging to help her body heal, but Joan refused because she had "prayed for God's will to be done." It never occurred to this devout lady that it might have been God's will for her to use the help available to her.

Acceptance of a personal faith does not mean passive fatalism. And neither does it mean pretending that everything is fine when you are hurting. I was not impressed with the man who told me that he fell flat on his back after slipping on an icy sidewalk. He said someone asked him if he was all right, and he responded, "I couldn't be better. I thank God for a safe landing."

That was a bit extreme. When you hurt, be honest. There's nothing wrong with saying, "I hurt." Acceptance means facing reality. Some would-be spiritual leaders seem to encourage unhealthy practices like denial. They teach people to ignore illness, pretending that everything is fine with them. Some even recommend thanking God for good health without acknowledging sickness of any kind. Such blindness will not stand alongside the Gethsemane faith of Jesus Christ, who prayed, "Father, if you are willing, take this cup from me; yet not my will, but yours be done." That is realism coupled with acceptance; that's determination to make things better, balanced with the resignation that accepts reality.

Healthy spirituality involves responsibility. I was asked recently, "Why teach methods of healing and prevention? When it's your time, you're going to die. There's nothing you can do about it, is there?" My answer was, yes, there is something you can do about it. Although many well-meaning people embrace this fatalistic concept, it's an idea that turns people into victims. And worse, it is not true.

Suppose we experiment to determine the effects of certain behaviors on health, assigning ten thousand people to two groups of five thousand each. One group smokes two packs of cigarettes per day, while the other abstains from smoking. If they live similar lifestyles, except for smoking, which group will, on the average, live longer? The nonsmokers, of course! They will live an average of eight to ten years longer. Is it strange that, on the average, "your time will come" earlier if you smoke than if you do not?

We can do the same experiment using exercise, nutrition, stress reduction, or positive emotional attitudes as variables and find significant differences in the life spans of two groups. We live longer, on the average, if we participate in an exercise program, maintain a balanced diet, control our stress, and have a positive outlook on life.

Don't seek to blame others for things over which you actually have control. In the Old Testament, Ezekiel writes: "'The fathers eat sour grapes, and the children's teeth are set on edge . . . [but] the soul who sins is the one who will die" (18:2-4). This is another way of saying "you reap what you sow."

Lifestyle clearly has an effect on general health and longevity. Healthy spirituality leaves room for personal responsibility and participation in its own health programs. In other words, "trust God, but tie up your camel."

Spiritually healthy people work to improve their health. Acceptance of your health situation doesn't mean you give up trying to improve your health. I worked very hard with Joan, the young cancer patient I mentioned earlier, trying to persuade her to get involved in her treatment program. But because of her misguided faith, she resisted all my attempts to help. Joan was expressing honest, but I think unhealthy, religious practice when she said, "I've prayed, and I believe God will heal me. I should not pursue any other avenues to healing." By limiting her options she was also limiting how God could heal her. She was looking for a dramatic, lightning-bolt type healing, and she overlooked the more ordinary miracles. Maybe God's chosen mode of healing were the resources he had provided for her. She chose not to use them, and she died shortly thereafter. There is no guarantee she would have lived longer, but she did not give life a full chance.

God gives us a boat and oars, but we have to do the rowing. I accept what is; that is the source of contentment. But I work to make life as good as it can be. The Apostle Paul expressed this idea in Philippians 4:11, in which he said he had learned to be content, no matter what!

Healthy spirituality involves peace and contentment. Peace and contentment play an important role in health. But peace and contentment are often misunderstood. Peace is an inner feeling that comes with acceptance—not passivity that turns a person into a victim, helpless to improve his or her life. Peace results from knowing you have the ability to make the best of your life and accepting the realities of your circumstances. Contentment is a choice.

Being content with what you have does not mean that you never leave a bad job, end a bad relationship, or seek to improve your life. It simply means you accept responsibility for your decision-making and your decisions. It means you have enough sense to recognize what you can do, doing what you can, then leaving your troubles to God. Contentment allows you to rest!

Making wise decisions about life is a source of peace, and healthy spirituality means participating in decision-making. A state of indecision and confusion brings turmoil. When you put off decisions you feel uncomfortable. When you have decisions to make, you're wise to gather as much information as you can and make a decision. Peace will follow the decision-making.

A woman was at a loss to know how to handle the troubles in her marriage. One day she showed up at my office with a smile on her face. She said, "Well, I have made a decision: I am going to wait until June. If things in the marriage haven't improved by then, I'm going to try a new strategy." I cannot predict the outcome of her marriage, but her health is better because she has made a decision about something major that was troubling her.

Healthy spirituality involves thanksgiving and love. A friend named Rolland Brown once told me that peace is turned on at a faucet we cannot reach. We reach the faucet that turns on thanksgiving, and then some other hand then turns on peace. I like his idea. Expressing gratitude for the blessings of God is part of healthy spirituality.

But perhaps the deepest and most powerful spiritual characteristic is love. Like most other aspects of spirituality, it's important to strive for balance in the area of love. You need to balance your love for self with love for others, love for life, and love for God. Just as you have the freedom to express personal faith, you have the freedom to express and accept love.

How important is love? It may be the most powerful force in your life. According to Bernie Siegel, feelings of love and being loved actually affect your body in measurable ways. Love lowers the levels of lactic acid, thereby reducing fatigue. Love raises the levels of endorphins, which make people less subject to pain. Love increases the responsiveness of white blood cells, which naturally protect people against colds and other infections. Love reduces the risk of heart attacks.

Feeling love even reduces the rate of accidents. Working husbands whose wives kiss them good-bye before work live longer than those who do not get kissed. It isn't the kiss, but the love that the kiss expresses that produces a healthy effect in their lives.

Love for others begins with an awareness that you are loved. Some people feel unworthy. They think they have to suffer cancer or some other problem in order to "deserve" love. This is *not true!* Jesus taught that we are to love our neighbors as we love ourselves. How do we love ourselves? One friend suggested that I could love myself by thinking of three or four things to do for someone I love and do something similar for myself.

We might write ourselves a nice note, buy ourselves a gift, take ourselves to dinner. We can be creative and extravagant in expressing love to ourselves, and then love others as we love ourselves.

Permit yourself to fall in love with life, with all of nature. Let walking in the park be a spiritual experience. Stop worrying about what anyone else would think, and be yourself. Let yourself love all creation freely. John Milton, the poet, wondered whether earth might be "but the shadow of Heaven." Perhaps this earth is only a shadow of reality and the true reality is far more real, more wonderful than anything we have ever imagined. That could really deepen our perception of this present world. C. S. Lewis seemed to agree with Milton. In his final Chronicles of Narnia book, *The Last Battle,* Narnia is ending, but her creatures move "further up and further in" to a Narnia that is more real, more meaningful, than the one they left.

It is the spiritual and healing experience of love that empowers us to let go of those things that block health and wholeness and cling to the things that anchor us to what is best in life.

When you begin to accept and experience love, especially and particularly unconditional love, you begin to learn some exciting things about life. Unconditional love does not have to be earned. It loves regardless of defects, and everyone has a right to it. It is the kind of love I experienced from my Grandmother Little. She loved me no matter what. She didn't approve of everything I did, but I never doubted her love. Her love was like God's love "with skin on."

I wish everyone could have that kind of love from someone. All of us are loved unconditionally by God. We'd all be healthier if we could comprehend that love in our physical and emotional lives. But none of us can receive love from others until we feel that we deserve and can have love. Christians believe that God loves us all, even when we are unlovely. "God so loved the world that he gave his one and only Son, that whoever believes in him shall not perish but have eternal life"

(John 3:16). If all Christians acted on that belief, we would all be healthier.

Healthy spirituality is grounded in hope. Once you grasp the fact that you are loved, you discover more easily a restoration and strengthening of hope. I will never forget the cancer patient who turned his treatment around and survived beyond all odds. I asked, "What was the most important and powerful thing you have learned in treatment?"

"That I have hope!" he said. Hope comes as a result of believing you have a chance to live and succeed. It is a result of goals and directions. It is the belief that the human being has been given a miraculous gift, a body that will often do whatever it takes to recover if we free it to work. Realistic hope recognizes the work to be done and accepts all the help it can get. Hope looks for help from God and from those people he puts into our lives to help us. Hope is a healing force, and it grows in the hothouse of love.

Love also reduces fear—a debilitating, costly emotion. Fear of rejection keeps you from reaching out to others. Fear of failure keeps you from trying anything new. Fear of pain prevents your crossing the threshold to peace. Fear of death obstructs life. Love and hope cast out fear. The Bible teaches that perfect love casts out all fear. When I am afraid, I remember arms of love around me, tender looks of love, words of encouragement and love, and I am not afraid.

To remind myself that I am loved, sometimes I slip back in my mind to early childhood experiences. One night, after I had been talking to some people about heart attacks, I felt a pain in my chest. I thought, "Maybe I'm having one myself. Maybe this is it!" I was alone. I wondered, "Should I write a final note? Should I try to call for help? Should I wait?" "Oh, God," I thought, "what if I'm dying?"

I was on the edge of panic when I realized my symptoms were not real. But my fear was. Then I remembered a childhood prayer that I prayed with my grandmother. It's the prayer I taught Andy in his hospital room: "Now I lay me down to sleep, I pray the Lord my soul to keep. If I should die before I wake, I pray the Lord my soul to take. God bless my family. Amen." I soon drifted off to sleep on memories of love that casts out fear.

Healthy Spirituality Is Free from False Guilt.
Love combats guilt, and who doesn't feel some guilt? Some guilt is deserved, and it has a purpose. We often resist temptation because we know what guilt a wrongful act will cause. Preventing us from wrongdoing and motivating us to do what's right are constructive uses for guilt.

Unfortunately, there are also several destructive uses for guilt. Some people use guilt to salve their consciences when they have misbehaved. "Well, yes," they tell themselves, "I lied, but I feel guilty. If I were not such a good person, I wouldn't feel guilty."

Some use guilt to make themselves miserable. But you can be forgiven for anything if you are truly sorry and honestly mean to do better. You can accept forgiveness of others as a gift. You can extend forgiveness to those who have hurt you. Those of us who have found personal forgiveness in the grace of Christ know the joy of being forgiven. We have every reason to forgive ourselves and others.

Withholding forgiveness and holding onto resentments can make you sick. Resentment is like a burr in your pocket. It sticks you every time you sit down, and by the time you give it to someone you "have it in for," its sharpness has been dulled on your own backside. Withholding forgiveness always hurts you more than it hurts anyone else.

If you are holding resentment, release it. Telephone the person you resent or write a letter. You don't have to become "bosom buddies." Just let go of the resentment. If you forgive real and imagined hurts you will free your own system to fight for your health.

I am thankful for every day of life. When I feel tense and worried, I sit down, take a deep breath, and list the things for which I am thankful. Counting my blessings nearly always results in an experience of peace and joy. Try it.

Are You Spiritually Healthy?

Peace and joy are those spiritual twins that energize life and health, and cure and prevent disease. How do you find them? Express your faith in God; dare to love; let go of fear, guilt, and despair; dare to hope; and express gratitude.

Joy and peace flow from invisible sources you cannot control, but you can reach love, forgiveness, and gratitude. Turn those emotions on, and the unseen hands of Another will turn on peace and joy.

Step Eight: Exercise Healthy Spirituality

Joy is vital to healthy living. When Walter Russell—author, philosopher, musician, and artist—called joy one of the five keys to success and the crowning key, he wasn't talking about the superficial appearance of the "hail fellow, well met with a smile," but of deep satisfaction and happiness that come from a sense of self-worth and self-respect. There is no deeper sense of joy than that which comes from respecting the way we live.

Healthy spirituality is never a matter of outward ritual or legalistic rule-following. It is certainly not limited to organizational or institutional religion, though it is frequently found there. True spirituality is a matter of the heart. It is healthy and healing. I know of no more valuable attitude for prevention and healing of disease than this kind of spirituality.

In my study of cancer patients, the longtime survivors said remarkable things to me about the power of spiritual strength.

"I used to feel ugly because of marks on my face," said one woman. "Now I laugh about them. When I start to get depressed, I pray and read the Bible. The health program you described helped me realize that cancer does not equal death. I am going to get a job to keep occupied instead of sitting."

This woman had learned to use her sense of humor, her joy of living. She had become an active participant in her own health care. She was trusting God and doing all she could to help herself. That is true spirituality.

I have suggested eight steps toward health and wholeness. I believe that none of them are more important than embracing a healthy spiritual faith.

Participating This Week

Build your spiritual health by taking time to look over the meditations for Step Eight at the back of this book. Time for reflective peace and quiet is good for your body and your spirit.

Chapter 11

The Last Word

There are some things that I believe strongly. As far as my experience goes, I *know* them. I know that people will be healthier if they practice regular relaxation. If relaxation is combined with regular deep breathing and periods of meditation on positive things, all the better. Relaxation does not hurt anyone. It helps. You will have a better chance of avoiding disease if you practice relaxation. Even when you are not sick, you are wise to practice relaxation daily. Two and a half years into his "three months of life," I asked Dave what had helped him most in the adjunct treatment program. "I'm more relaxed about life," he said. "I practice relaxation with an audio tape three times a day. I'm able to flow with life. That is one very important benefit to me."

I know that picturing health through images and word pictures will help people get well and stay healthier. I sometimes imagine myself running or shooting a basketball when I am sixty-five years old. I suspect that when I'm sixty-five I will imagine doing those things at seventy or seventy-five. That image is healthy because, in order to make it come true, I will have to be healthy. I imagine myself trim—a lean, mean machine. That picture implies that my diet will be good and my exercise sufficient. Picture health in whatever way works for you. Use your imagination—wake it up and dust it off. Our dreams have a way of coming true. I have written it this way, "I dreamed a dream and set it asail. I dreamed a dream and watched it fail. But faith will find a way to win. I just dreamed my dream again." I am an optimist, so even if a dream failed temporarily, I'd dream it again. I imagine. I envision. I dream of health and wholeness.

I know that exercise—at least a moderate aerobic exercise program—helps people stay healthy. Since the exercise craze of the late sixties we've seen a steady decline in the incidence of strokes and heart attacks, according to Dr. Kenneth Cooper. He says that the average age of heart-attack victims is on the rise. Your body functions better when you exercise it than when you let it atrophy in front of the television.

I know that participating in your own health care is better for you than assuming the role of a victim. The patients with whom I work consistently affirm the importance of participation. They unanimously echo the words of a breast cancer patient: "In addition to relaxation and goal setting, one of the most important things I've learned in the adjunct treatment program is that I am involved in my own health care. It gives me a sense of strength and at least some measure of control."

We have been so afraid of inducing guilt by telling people that they participate in their disease, and thus in their health, that we kill them with kindness. We hurt diabetics if we tell them they have no responsibility for their diet. We damage patients with oat-cell carcinoma of the lungs when we pretend that they didn't do it to themselves by smoking. Holding in anger and anxiety and dealing inappropriately with such emotions is unhealthy. Drinking alcohol injures the alcoholic.

No one directly chooses to have cancer, high blood pressure, strokes, ulcers, heart attacks, and other illnesses. But we certainly choose the lifestyles that lead to these problems. The good news is that, since we are involved in sickness, we can be involved in getting well and staying well. It is healthy to be an active participant in your own health care. Read about health. Ask questions of your doctors. Believe in yourself and become an active participant in your own wellness and wholeness.

I know that a clear and specific philosophy and healthy religious faith have beneficial effects on your health. Dave continued answering the question about benefits from our adjunct treatment program: "I now have a more clear conviction about God," he said. "I believed in God before I began this program, but it was a kind of general faith. Now I have a personal relationship with God. That has helped me." Never be ashamed of your spiritual life. It gives depth to your existence and helps you to stay well.

I know that a sense of purpose is healthy. Life has to go somewhere; the direction is up to you. Set goals. There is magnetic and energizing power in purpose, in goals. If I get on a plane, I want to know where it is going. And on this trip through life, I want to know where I'm going, so I set goals. Goals give me direction and a purpose. I encourage my clients to set goals and, when they begin to achieve them, to re-set them. Always keep something in front of you that is worth living for, and maybe you *will* live!

I know that having fun is healthy. Laughing is relaxing. Laughing is energizing. Laughing is a painkiller. You'll live longer and be healthier if you have fun. Enjoy life! Read joke books, view funny movies, whatever it takes. Find a way to have fun. I listened to a child's view of some of our history. One child said about the Reformation: "Martin Luther was nailed to the door of the church at Wittenburg. That later led to his death, and he remained dead to this day." I laughed, of course. Remember that life is too important to take seriously. Laugh a little. It's healthy.

I know that positive attitudes and thinking are healthy. Norman Vincent Peale is right. There is power in positive thinking. I am not an unrealistic Pollyanna skipping through life. Pain is real to me, sickness is real, sorrow is real. But so is comfort, so is wellness, so is joy. Since I live in my own thoughts, I will make my home in the land of positives. I choose to think positively, and I believe that is healthy. Accentuate the positives!

I know that a high-fiber, low-fat, regulated diet is healthy. You are what you think and what you eat. Some people are great big negative cheeseburgers. I want to be a positive bowl of mixed fruit or an apple. Proper diet reduces cholesterol, shrinks ulcers, and eliminates swelling hemorrhoids. Proper diets that include lots of fruit and vegetables are healthy. If you eat right, you live longer and stay healthier.

I know that love and encouragement are healthy. Fall in love with life, with your family, with God, with the world. When you are in love, you feel better. I don't mean only romantic love. I mean love that cares about life and people. Lucy, from the comic strip *Peanuts,* says, "Charlie Brown, you blockhead, I love the world. It's the people I can't stand." That won't work. Love is encouragement, encouragement for yourself and for others. Encourage others—it's energizing. *No one ever died from an overdose of encouragement.*

Above all, I am certain that hope is healthy. Do not be afraid to hope. Hope ties it all together. If you come to the end of your rope, tie a knot in it!

Relax every day!
Picture health!
Exercise!
Participate in your health care!
Believe in something beyond yourself!
Set goals!
Have fun!
Be positive!
Eat right!
Choose love and encouragement!
Hang on to your hope!
Here's to your health!

Appendix A

Daily Thoughts on the Eight Steps

We can change, but we cannot change without real commitment and effort. Simply reading a book or attending one seminar won't bring about real change. Truly changing beliefs and lifestyles takes persistent effort—and not just for a week or two. It will probably take about a year.

Do you believe change is worth the investment of your time and effort? I believe that it is—even in dollars and cents. With the rising costs of health care, isn't the best solution for every person to take better care of his or her health? Prevention of even some disease would immediately bring down the cost of medical care and, at the same time, would raise the quality of life for those who prevent disease.

The eight steps described in this book are designed not only to help us heal, but also to help us prevent disease. The material in this section is designed to supplement the preceding chapters. Each step toward health is supplemented by seven thoughts or meditations. If you really want to change, these will be a great ally in your quest.

To get the most from these exercises:

1. *Read, stop, think.* Read each meditation, then stop and think about what you have read. To meditate literally means "to mull over." So ponder, reflect, study, and think. If something in the meditation sparks a memory of something you read earlier in this book, take the time to review that material. This isn't a race; there's no pressure to finish your time of meditation quickly. So take your time.
2. *Write it down.* A notepad and pen make great learning tools. As I meditate, I take time to write down my thoughts: What things really apply to me or my situation?
3. *Make a plan.* As I discover insights that apply to me, I develop a plan of action. Those insights are no good to me unless they take on the solid form of a goal.

Because there are eight steps, the meditations take eight weeks. Make a commitment to follow through for all the weeks required to finish these meditations. This is an important step toward accomplishing your goal to get well and stay well. It's directly up to you.

Week 1

Thoughts for Step One: Choose to Live

Day 1: Choose to Get Started

You want to be healthier. You want to live a long and high-quality life. It is the right thing to do, but where and how do you get started?

You start where you are—with your present needs. Do you need to take more responsibility for the way you use your time? Do you need to take some time for yourself? Do you need to spend more time with someone you love? You start by taking charge of the areas that are important to you. The important thing is to start.

Some people have to begin exercising by taking a single step. One person may start an exercise program simply by walking around a room or raising a head off the pillow. When I am too tired for exercise or am tempted not to exercise, I remember a promise I made to a friend who was confined to a wheelchair. I said, "I will run for both of us." I do something he wishes he could do. I run.

Think about this: The great saints of God began their spiritual pilgrimages by reading one word of devotional material and by praying one prayer. They started. The greatest athletes began by lifting a small amount of weight or running a slow jog. But they started.

We do not grow or improve without getting started. This principle is spiritual in nature. We cannot begin a spiritual journey without taking the first step—an open expression of our faith. This principle is also physical in nature. Training begins with the first step, whether it's jogging or any other form of exercise.

There is a passage in the Bible (Ecclesiastes 3:1-8) that says there is a time for everything. The time for us to begin a program of growth and improvement is now. Write in your journal or notebook, "I have started. That is my choice."

Think of actual, concrete things you will do to take strides toward health. Set a time, and get started. Choose to begin!

Day 2: Choice Is the Beginning of Excellence

One of the greatest discoveries of my life was the discovery that I have choices. I have choices about almost everything. For example, I do not "lose" my temper. I choose my temper and use my temper. When someone cuts me off in traffic I make a decision. Many people act as if there is no decision; they follow a set pattern for reaction. But each person can ask, "How do I want to respond? What results do I want?" It may be difficult, but anyone can begin to choose his or her emotions and actions.

Another proof of the fact that we choose our responses is found in the teaching of Jesus Christ to "love your enemies." He knew we could choose how we would respond to others.

When my oldest son, B.J., was in his early teens he would occasionally do something that I disapproved of. Knowing my desire to control my emotions and act instead of react, B.J. learned to ask me, "Dad, are you going to choose to be upset about this?"

Sometimes the answer was "Yes!" But there were times when his question reminded me of my power to control and choose my responses, and I could choose not to be upset.

It is the awareness of choice that paves the way for excellence. If you don't know you have choices or if you ignore your choices, you are doomed to go through life responding to every stimulus you confront. Life will happen to you, when you could be happening to life. So take control.

Do you choose to live today? That is a conscious choice—one that will influence your habits. Are you going to exercise today? The choice is yours. Are you going to be angry, sad, glad, or loving today? Emotional responses can be chosen. The choice is yours.

Choose to make choices!

Day 3: Take Responsibility for Life

There are some universal constants, and some of these natural laws will nag or comfort us all through our lives. One law that does both is the law of sowing and reaping: "You will reap what you sow."

This law is sometimes comforting. I am pleased that when I go through the discipline of regular aerobic exercise, I will someday reap the benefits of better cardiovascular condition. But the law of sowing and reaping nags at me sometimes, too. For example, it bothers me that the evidence of my eating habits will show up in my bloodstream.

Whether you like it or not, the fact remains that you are responsible for your condition, and your condition is directly related to the law of sowing and reaping. You can deny it, but it will stubbornly decree that you are responsible for yourself.

In the Bible, the apostle Paul writes: "Do not be deceived: God cannot be mocked. A man reaps what he sows" (Galatians 6:7). Self-deception is self-defeating. Can you remember a time in your life when you deceived yourself? Have you ever said, "One more won't hurt me?" If you can remember self-deception, write an example in your notebook. Call it by name and do not let it dupe you again.

A man once said that he sowed wild oats and then "prayed for crop failure." We all know he might not get what he's asking for. Life just doesn't work that way. Here is a wonderful admonition to ponder:

Sow a thought,
Reap a deed.
Sow a deed,
Reap a character.

You are responsible for who you are and what you are. Today you are reaping all that you planted in the past, and tomorrow you will reap what you plant today.

Some might accuse me of trying to make people feel guilty. Indeed, I do not intend for anyone to feel guilty about his or her lifestyle unless there is good reason. But by the same token, is it wise to never mention the relationship between smoking and lung cancer because a smoker who has lung cancer might feel guilty? Even at that risk I think we must get information out to those who continue to run the risk. Is it wise to never mention the relationship between driving drunk and fatal accidents? Is it wise never to mention the relationship between eating 50,000 (a slight exaggeration) calories of fat and clogged arteries or heart disease? I have seen too many obese ministers pointing fingers at others' sins, and I have helped to bury too many family and friends not to mention these facts. It is time to stop blaming everything around us and start assuming some personal responsibility.

Choose to take responsibility!

Day 4: Be a Participant

I once knew two men who had serious heart conditions. Their conditions were so serious that they were not even candidates for transplants. Gene's condition was worse, but neither man was expected to live a full year.

Joe did very little. He sat around a lot. He quit working and never played at all after his diagnosis. He rarely even walked around.

But Gene exercised faithfully. He kept on at his job as an insurance salesman (he even sold me an insurance policy that first year). He played—a lot. We even played catch in his back yard.

Within eight months, Joe was dead. Gene lived a high-quality life and died seven years later while taking a bath. Was the difference simply coincidental? I don't think so.

There are no absolute guarantees, but it does seem that those who actively participate in life live longer and higher-quality lives. The biblical book of Galatians teaches, "Let us not become weary in doing good, for at the proper time we will reap a harvest if we do not give up" (6:9).

In communicating, physical conditioning, relating, creating, and living our faith, intention alone means nothing. Doing means everything. A writer friend once told me, "The desire to write not followed by writing is the desire not to write." The desire to do anything, not followed by doing that thing is the desire not to do it.

Is there something you have been thinking of doing for a long time but just have never gotten around to? Write about it in your notebook, make a goal, and then do it.

Choose to participate!

Day 5: The Secret Is Responsible Action

One of the secrets of life is that what we receive from life—in all areas, including wellness and character—will depend on the quality and quantity of our own contributions. Even in our spiritual lives, our faith depends on our decision to accept God's free gift of grace. This is another way of saying, "What goes around, comes around."

I have often heard people say that they are waiting for their "ship to come in." And I wonder, have they sent any out? How do people "send out ships"? They begin by considering what they want to receive. If you want a healthy body, the way to "send out a ship" is to eat healthy foods, exercise, rest, reduce stress, and spend time in meditation daily. (Care for the body is also a spiritual service to God, according to Romans 12:1.)

It's a simple truth: you must take responsibility for your own health and wholeness—both physically and spiritually. No one cares more about your health than you do. If you do not take care of your own habits and lifestyle, then who will?

The balance between responsibility and blame is sometimes a difficult one to maintain. The difficulty does not, however, excuse us. You must still accept responsibility for yourself if you want to be a healthier person.

My experience in working with cancer patients for the last twenty years has clearly convinced me that those who accept responsibility and live responsibly live longer and higher-quality lives.

Choose to take responsible action.

Day 6: Pay the Price

Bruce Larson has written a book titled *There's a Lot More to Health than Not Being Sick*. More than the absence of disease, health is the presence of zest, joy, power, hope, and enthusiasm. These characteristics exist only in the lives of people who have "response-ability." These are the people who acknowledge the ability to respond to the demands of life.

Responsibility is a very close relative of accountability. To me this means that all of us are accountable for ourselves. Paul writes in Romans 14:12 that "each of us will give an account of himself to God."

When was the last time something went wrong in your life? Whom did you blame for it? Make a note of the situation and honestly examine it. Were there ways you contributed to the problem? You have much more power to solve problems when you honestly acknowledge responsibility. Winston Churchill once said, "Responsibility is the price of greatness." It is also the price of health, strong relationships, and personal growth. Are you willing to pay that price?

Mentally, you largely become what you think, watch, and read. Physically, in many ways you become what you eat. The Chinese have a proverb (they have proverbs for almost everything) that says, "Day by day, we write our own destiny, for we become what we do." You are responsible. Accepting that responsibility is a small price to pay for the kind of health that goes beyond the absence of lifestyle-related disease to the kind of energy that makes life exciting.

Choose to pay the price!

Day 7: Keep on Keeping on

As the pastor of a small country church, I was once given some wonderful advice by an old deacon named Mr. Jaynes. I was frustrated with the lack of support given to the church by its members. Discouraged, I went to Mr. Jaynes with my woes. After I finished complaining, I asked, "What can I do?"

The old man grinned knowingly, "Well, young man, you can just keep on keeping on." That was his advice. Over the years I've found that he summed things up very well. Getting started will mean nothing if you don't keep on. There will be times when hanging in there will be a major challenge—days of grief and pain when you will want to quit. The challenge then is just to put one foot in front of the other and keep going.

You'll find there are plenty of excuses for turning back from your commitments. Marriages are sometimes hard. Medical treatment programs are often hard. The pain of rejection or physical condition may make you feel like quitting. Keep going! Even when there are tears, keep putting one foot in front of the other. We see God most clearly through the prism of our tears.

Write in your notebook, "I will not quit. I have started, and I will keep on."

Choose to keep going!

Week 2

Thoughts for Step Two: Adopt Healthy Beliefs

Day 1: Mind and Body

Some people cannot see beyond their noses. Very few people can see a thing beyond what they already believe. What people believe determines what they are able to see and do. The idea that belief is related to health and wholeness, and even to the ability to get well, may be a new concept to you. But evidence is accumulating that there is no separation between mind and body. What happens to the body happens in the mind, and what happens in the mind happens to the body.

This is new thinking for most of us. We would do best, however, if we do not hold on to all our old belief systems. "No one sews a patch of unshrunk cloth on an old garment, for the patch will pull away from the garment, making the tear worse. Neither do men pour new wine into old wineskins. If they do, the skins will burst, the wine will run out and the wineskins will be ruined. No, they pour new wine into new wineskins, and both are preserved" (Matthew 9:16-17). Often when we try to fit new ideas into old belief systems, those belief systems have to break. Are you willing to break your old thought systems? At least I hope you will leave room for the development of new beliefs.

Thoughts for Step Two

What you think about your own body's ability to heal itself; what you believe about the effect of exercise; what you believe about the importance of nutrition; and *what you believe, period,* will determine your ability to accept and use new ideas about health and wholeness.

Over the years I have been forced to change a lot of beliefs. I'm not ashamed of this. I realize that means my mind is open to accepting new data. At one time I believed no human being could ever run a mile in under four minutes. Then, when that happened, I believed no human being could run a mile in under three minutes and fifty seconds. It was impossible. When that happened, I changed my mind again. I now believe that no one knows how fast a human being will be able to run a mile.

Can you list in your notebook two or three beliefs you have changed?

Do you believe that your beliefs can help you prevent disease? Do you believe that your beliefs can help your body heal? Remember that your beliefs either free you or limit you in becoming a stronger and healthier person.

Believe!

Day 2: Believing Is Doing

There is one very powerful belief about which I no longer have any doubts. That is, "No one behaves consistently at a level inconsistent with his or her self-concept." What does this mean? It means that what a person believes about himself or herself fairly well determines that person's performance, motivation, creativity, spiritual growth, and, to a large degree, health. I've seen multitudes of examples of this.

You've probably heard of the numerous studies indicating that a child's performance in school is influenced by what that young person believes about his or her ability. Remember Phil, the baseball player who hit only one home run in his first season? The second year he hit twenty-six home runs. A major difference—and all as a result of his self-concept. He said about his higher performance, "Last year I didn't know I could hit home runs!"

Sometimes a person fails to get well or to resist disease because he or she didn't know it was possible to get well and resist disease! Our bodies tend to do what we think they will do. When we know they are strong, they tend to hit home runs.

My grandmother used to tell a story about an old woman who heard that faith could move mountains. She stood at the base of a mountain, closed her eyes and prayed, "Mountain, be moved." Then she opened her eyes and said, "Just as I expected. It's still here."

This woman obviously didn't have the faith in the first place. Her unbelief proves a point: It's not what we say we believe, but what we really believe that determines our reality. When Jesus healed two blind men, he said to them, "According to your faith will it be done to you" (Matthew 9:29).

Write yourself a note that says, "I am not going to miss good health due to a lack of positive beliefs. I will build positive beliefs about my body."

Believe!

Day 3: Take What Is and Make the Most of It

You have the right to take what is—your present circumstance or situation—and make the most of it without complaining. The apostle Paul said about himself: "I have learned the secret of being content in any and every situation" (Philippians 4:12). Those who indulge in what I call "greener grassing" are some of the most miserable people in the world. They think they would be happier with a different husband or wife. They think they'd be happier if they lived in another neighborhood. The root of their problem is that they think their unhappiness, and thus their happiness, is external—depending on circumstances around them. That is not true!

Happiness and unhappiness are inside jobs. We make ourselves unhappy when we look at others and think we would be happier with what they have. But the happiest and healthiest people in the world are those who have decided to take what they have and make the very most of it.

My dad used to say there were two ways to be wealthy. The first would be to have enough money to buy anything you want. The second would be to want what you have enough money to buy. He claimed to be wealthy because he had learned to want what he could afford.

As trite as it may sound, it is healthy to take the lemons life hands us and make lemonade. It is healthy to take the stumbling stones and turn them into stepping stones. It is healthy to take problems and turn them into opportunities.

When you adopt a mindset that enables you to take what is and make the most of it, you reduce your stress, become happier, and become healthier. Make this commitment to yourself and write it out: "I will take what I have and make the very most of it that I can."

Make the most of your circumstances!

Day 4: The Prism of Perception

Every event, experience, conversation, and sight is filtered through the "prism of perception." A prism filters light so that anything viewed through it appears to be different. Everything we encounter is filtered through our internal beliefs to determine what we perceive as reality. It doesn't matter what the true facts are; each of us lives in the world of our perceptions.

I have long loved the comment of Paul to Titus: "To the pure, all things are pure, but to those who are corrupted and do not believe, nothing is pure. In fact, both their minds and consciences are corrupted" (Titus 1:15). An event may be neutral in and of itself, but we give meaning to it through our internal system of beliefs.

Sickness has physical properties and it is certainly not *all* just "in your mind," but there is a lot of it there. *You can make yourself less effective or more effective in dealing with sickness through your perceptions.*

The same illness will hang on for weeks in one person while another will throw it off within a matter of days. Part of the reason for that may be genetic inheritance. Part of the reason may be general physical condition. But more than you'd expect, perceptions, beliefs, and attitudes play a role. Perceive yourself to be a healthy person. Your body will fight for your health every day.

Perceive yourself healthy!

Day 5: Good Happens to You

One of my key beliefs is that everything works for good. I believe this is healthy. It certainly is a spiritual truth. Scripture teaches, "We know that in all things God works for the good of those who love him, who have been called according to his purpose" (Romans 8:28). Does that include you?

This does not mean that everything that happens to us *is* good. There are a lot of rotten things that happen in this world. Life is unfair. No one can deny the reality of bad things. To deny such realities would be a form of mental illness. But I am suggesting that if we choose to, we can find some good result in everything that happens to us.

The mindset that "everything works for good" enables you to look for the good. And finding the good can ease the pain of whatever is happening in your world. That is what God intends for his people.

Children are wonderful teachers. One child who had cancer believed he had cancer so he could learn how to be a doctor when he grew up. He found hope and dreams in the presence of sickness. He found the good in a difficult circumstance.

Can you identify something from your own life that initially appeared to be a terrible thing, but in retrospect you found some good in it? Make a note about it in your notebook. If you can't remember something from your own life, think of something you've seen work this way in a friend's life, or use your imagination to envision a scenario in which this would be true. Taking note of these circumstances is good practice. Practice looking for the good. Tell yourself repeatedly, "I believe everything works for good in my life." This is a healthy thought.

Look for the good!

Day 6: You Have Personal Worth

You have as much worth and value as anyone in all the world. You don't have to earn it. You don't have to prove it. It's yours because you are a human being. You have as much worth and value as anyone in the world, and so do I.

Jesus taught that you are so valued individually that the very hairs on your head are numbered (Luke 12:7). When you begin to recognize your worth and value, you begin to take better care of yourself.

I spoke at a grade school recently, explaining to the students that they all were of equal value and worth. I then gave them a test. I asked, "Who is more important, a doctor or a patient?"

"Neither," they responded. "Everyone is equal."

"That's right," I agreed. "And who is more important, a teacher or a student?"

"Neither," they beamed. "Everyone is equal."

"All right, who is more important, a parent or a child?"

They yelled, "Neither! Everyone is equal."

I figured they'd gotten the point, but I asked one more question: "Who is more important, boys or girls?"

"Girls!" screamed the girls.

"Boys!" yelled the boys.

We all have blind spots and prejudices. Are there some people you consider your equals and others you consider not so important? Don't let yourself get away with such prejudices. Make a note to yourself: "I will make a conscious effort to recognize the basic value of every human being, including myself."

If I am important, so are you. We both have worth and value.

Remember your worth and value!

Day 7: Hope

There is no such thing as false hope. There is only hope. Hope is the energy that keeps us going in the darkest hours of life. It enables us to live in expectation of seeing the morning sun.

It is written of Abraham that "against all hope, Abraham in hope believed . . . without weakening in his faith" (Romans 4:18-19). Abraham had a specific hope—the promise of a son. But we also have received promises from God, and there are certainly times when each of us is called upon to hope "against hope." I do not believe such hope is false.

Norman Cousins wrote, "People tell me not to offer hope unless I know hope to be real, but I don't know enough to say that hope can't be real. I'm not sure anyone knows enough to deny hope." I often talk with those who are ill or hurting, and I never ask them to lie to themselves. I try never to lie to them. But I do ask people to hold on to their hope. I tell them that hope is always real. I believe that.

As a positive emotion, hope gives rise to health and wholeness. So speak to yourself in positive terms. Use the language of hope. The principle of hope applies to financial situations that seem impossible. It applies to relationships that seem broken. It applies to illnesses that seem

Thoughts for Step Two

incurable. There are few, if any, diseases from which someone has not recovered. There is always hope.

Promise yourself and write down, "I will never stop hoping." Hope is energy for wholeness.

Never stop hoping!

Week 3

Thoughts for Step Three: Find Meaning

Day 1: Find Meaning in Your Life

Is there a point to life? You will have to answer that question for yourself. No one can answer for you or for anyone else. Personally, I believe the point to my life is to trust in God and make a positive difference in this world.

Another writer said his purpose was to love people and teach them how to love. Management writer Stephen Covey suggests taking the time to write a mission statement for yourself. Have you ever done that? If not, try it now. Write a clear statement of what you consider your purpose in life to be.

Such an exercise is helpful to your health—in fact, it's vital to both mental and physical health. Direction in life raises your energy level. When you have a sense of direction you will feel the focus. It is draining to live in a state of confusion or ambiguity about life. Surely it is apparent that when your energy levels are high you feel better physically. That energy is required to maintain good health.

The healthiest person who ever lived had a clear and precise mission in life. He knew his purpose. Jesus said the purpose in life is to "seek first his kingdom [God's] and his righteousness, and all these things [necessities] will be given to you as well" (Matthew 6:33).

Take time to write a mission statement for yourself. It doesn't have to be perfect; it just has to be yours. You can always rewrite it.

Your life has meaning.

Day 2: Life Has Meaning

I believe that my life has meaning. I believe in the larger purpose of God for my life, and I want to cast myself as part of God's plan.

Believing that life has purpose is a source of power for daily living. In fact, there are times when the belief that there is a reason for living is the only thing that keeps us going.

The most quoted people on this topic are Victor Frankl and Rollo May, both of whom were in the Nazi concentration camps during World War II. These men have taught us from their experiences a great deal about the power to live. Both were determined that the Nazis would never deprive them of their freedom to give meaning to their lives. Frankl said that there were times when he felt more free than his captors because he retained his freedom to give meaning to his own life.

Rollo May eventually came to the conclusion that freedom is "the ability to pause between the stimulus and the response and in that pause choose the response." If the prison camp experience was the stimulus, the response was to give meaning to life, even in those conditions.

It is a great problem in the world that there is so much loss of individual meaning. Some seem to try to replace meaning with a selfish focus on personal rights. No amount of focus on individual rights will replace individual meaning.

I have determined that I will find substance for my life. If nothing else, I will find people who are suffering and help to ease their pain. There is meaning to my life. No one can take that from me.

What is the most meaningful thing you have done today? This week? Ever? Think about your answers. Write them down and reflect on them. Vow to become conscious of purpose in daily life.

Your life has meaning.

Day 3: Discover Your Meaning

Oliver Wendell Holmes said, "What lies behind us and what lies before us are tiny matters compared to what lies within us." Jesus Christ tells us what is within us. He said, "The kingdom of God is within you" (Luke 17:21). I think that part of what he meant is that we have within us our own meaning, planted like a seed waiting to grow. All that remains is for us to discover that seed and begin to nurture it in faith by asking, searching, and continuing in a relationship with God.

One way to find meaning is to ask yourself how you would like to be remembered. Think about it. The answer is within you. A cancer patient recently told me that she asked herself that question. The answer was that she wants to be remembered as someone who cared. She is finding meaning in life by doing things for others. She calls friends who are ill and offers to help them. She invites lonely acquaintances out for lunch. She finds a way to care, simple ways that give meaning (see Matthew 25).

Meaning does not have to be dramatic; it just has to be yours. Often it is found in asking yourself what you really enjoy doing. That "seed" inside you seeks expression. When you ask the right question, the answer is ready.

You usually know more than you realize. Frequently you can find answers inside yourself if you just take the time to seek. You might discover meaning by asking three questions and writing down your answers to them. Here they are:

How do I want to be remembered?
What would I enjoy doing with my life?
What would give me a sense of satisfaction in life?

When you answer these questions you may well discover the meaning that is within yourself.

Your life has meaning.

Day 4: Ease Pain

I believe the greatest sign that the kingdom of God has come into the world is the alleviation of human suffering. To me, there could be no greater good accomplished in life than to help ease people's pain. I find meaning in attempting to find ways to alleviate the suffering of my fellow human beings. For, me there is meaning in listening to a frightened cancer patient talk about his fears. If I can hold the patient's hand and offer words of encouragement, my life has meaning.

Think about it. Have you ever had the experience of easing someone's pain? How did you feel when that happened?

Have you ever needed to have someone alleviate your suffering? If so, what do you think about that person right now?

There is no scarcity of pain. People suffer pain ranging from simple headaches to facing terminal illness and the loss of life. You don't have to go on a crusade to find people in distress. All you have to do is become aware of the trials in the lives of people around you and make some practical effort to reduce their discomfort.

It may be that you will find meaning in lots of different things, but if you have not found personal meaning yet you might find it in this action: Alleviate human suffering wherever it can be found.

Your life has meaning.

Day 5: Success and Meaning

I believe we all want to be successful. It is just hard to know what that means. Some set a monetary goal as a standard for success. I find that to be a little empty. When I looked into my own heart, I decided that success for me meant "to find ways to alleviate human suffering and live with as much joy as possible in that process." For me this is consistent with Christian teaching. Jesus certainly alleviated human suffering wherever he went. He also taught his followers to live with abundance.

My father never wrote a mission statement for himself, but he did have a clear notion as to what it meant to live successfully. About a year before he died, I recorded a conversation with him. In that conversation he said, "Bill, some people measure their success in life by how much money they earned. I never did that. I measured my success by how much fun I had. I have had a lot of fun. There is not much about my life that I would change."

Now, I know that life is a lot more than fun. That might not be a measure of success for many, but there is nothing wrong with adding that dimension to your own life.

Success and meaning for me are in alleviating human suffering, pleasing God, and spreading as much joy as I can, while remaining true to what I believe I am supposed to be.

Think about this: Success in life may be measured by the ability to take whatever comes and make the most of it (Philippians 4:11-13).

Day 6: Values

One way to find meaning in life is to live according to your own real values. When you decide what is important to you, you are wise to avoid compromise.

If family is important, then determine to set aside time to spend with them. Let nothing change that. Love is a four-letter word often spelled T-I-M-E. If you think you are spending a lot of time with your family, check yourself. For the next two weeks keep a record of the time you spend in family activities. I mean family activities that involve interaction. This excludes time in front of the television. You may be surprised at how little real interaction goes on between you and the ones you love.

If personal faith is important to you, make that known by the way you spend your time and by the direction of your conversations.

The point is that you find meaning when you live according to your own values. You should not be reluctant to express those values. Honesty, work, faith, family, service, friendship, love, generosity, and kindness have not fallen out of favor.

A Greek philosopher said that happiness is found through living your life in such a way that you respect what you are doing. Meaning is found in the same way. Live according to your own values. They give meaning to you.

Your life has meaning.

Day 7: Lost Meaning Is Lost Life

While I was doing a radio show with my friend Jim White, a caller phoned to ask for help. He believed his physical condition (fainting spells) was more emotional than physical. He said he felt useless on his job and that his coworkers saw him as useless, too. The only possible meaning to his job was that he earned a living, and this was not enough to satisfy his desire to mean something. He was forty-nine and still lived with his mother—not because she needed him but because he needed the security of being there with her.

There was an empty sound in his voice. "My life is over," he said. He had given up.

I asked him what would have made his life different and better. He answered, "If I had been kicked out of the house when I was twenty-one it would have been better for me." He had learned to rely on his parents for his security and, after forty-nine years, he was afraid to leave.

He was asking me to tell him how he could find meaning in his life. He knew that without meaning there was no life. I tried to help, but he just couldn't believe his life was worth anything. There is hope for this man; he just has to accept responsibility for himself and get moving. It would have been easier at twenty-one, but he can still do it at forty-nine.

How about you? What are you selling your life for? Do you feel that it's too late for you? I don't believe it is too late. Start now to find and give meaning to your life. There is meaning in living.

Your life has meaning.

Week 4

Thoughts for Step Four: Control Stress

Day 1: Relax

The first step to preventing disease and empowering the healing process for most people is relaxation. Have you ever said, "I just never seem to have time for me. It's impossible to drop any activities. I just wish the world would stop." If you have, you're not the only one. Many contemporary people could say the same thing. Such a lifestyle is best described as "lowering empty buckets into empty wells and pulling them up as fast as we can, empty." That kind of living is damaging to your health.

There is little question that stress is a major health problem. Stress seems to retard the immune system, and prolonged stress is a predictor of illness. If you want to prevent disease in your life, you must learn to manage stress effectively.

One skill that will help you manage stress is the skill of relaxation—and it is a skill. Skills can be learned. There are several ways to learn relaxation. You could use a relaxation tape. Or you could look into progressive relaxation techniques. (This technique is outlined in the Guidebook for Cancer Patients in Appendix B of this book).

Read material that helps you relax. The Bible teaches that we can enter into the "rest" of the Lord (Hebrews 4:9-11). What do you suppose that means? Write your answer and think about it.

Invest at least ten minutes twice a day in practicing relaxation.

You can learn to relax.

Day 2: Free From Anxiety

Relaxation and faith have a lot in common. Faith in what is good and faith in God can reduce your anxieties and enable you to relax. The great apostle Paul wrote, "Do not be anxious about anything, but in everything, by prayer and petition with thanksgiving, present your requests to God. And the peace of God, which transcends all understanding, will guard your hearts and your minds in Christ Jesus" (Philippians 4:6-7). He goes on to ask people to think about things that are true, good, pure, and respected (v. 8).

Some people who read this say that of course Paul could say this to readers in the simple world of the first century, but things are different, more complicated now. I say, it's not the world that has changed so much. It's people who have changed.

You will always have to deal with pain, sorrow and loss. Those things are part of life. But that does not mean you will always have to live with anxiety or depression. Simple faith and focusing on what is best in your life and world will enable you to walk through it all in peace.

Most depression and anxiety are unnecessary, and it is always destructive to one's health. A few years ago, a song captured the public's imagination with its simple theme: "Don't Worry, Be Happy." The concept is over-simplified, but is nevertheless headed in the right direction.

Relaxation is more than an exercise or physical skill, though it is that, too. Relaxation is also a matter of attitude, a matter of belief, a matter of focus.

I find that relaxation and peace come easier for me when I begin times of meditation and rest by thinking of things for which I am thankful.

Try it. Take a deep breath and after slowly releasing it begin naming things for which you are grateful. You will probably begin to feel a sense of peace deep inside. Be a grateful person. It is relaxing.

You can learn to relax.

Day 3: Mellow Out

I heard a cardiologist say that we create the conditions conducive to heart attacks because we struggle too much with the small stuff. Then he added, "It's *all* small stuff." He was right. When it comes down to life or death, usually the annoyances that pester us from day to day begin to look pretty petty.

I was thankful for his comments. That was an idea I could live with! It reminds me not to take myself and my activities so seriously.

Another way I help myself relax is that I tell myself I am mellow. Try it. Say to yourself: "I am mellow." Even the words feel relaxed. Mellow means "laid back." It means "not strung out." Even if you are not totally mellow right now you can begin by just saying the words. It is hard to maintain a rigid attitude while saying, "I am mellow."

I also attempt to maintain some balance in my life by using bumper-sticker philosophies. These are easy for me to remember, and in stressful situations they bring a smile to my face and make me relax a little. These little mottoes keep me mellow. Stack as many of them as you can into your own memory bank.

"Stay in the flow." That is a little motto that comes to mind when I begin rushing too much. I first heard it from a speech given by Robert Eliot a few years ago. He said, "When you can't fight and you can't flee, then flow."

I put those words and other mottoes on audio tape and play them for myself as I drive to work some days. Try it.

You can learn to relax.

Day 4: Chill out

Young people have a wonderful way with words. One of my favorites is, "Chill out." The short form is simply, "Chill." When my youngest son, Russ, hears tension in my voice during a conversation he says, "Chill out, Dad" or "Chill, dude." As long as he says it with a smile I can respond well. I know he's right. It's always better to "chill."

Try using his expression. Say to yourself, "I am chilled out." Repeat it fifteen or twenty times a day for the next week and see what feelings follow. I think you will be pleased, if not chilled.

Here are some short phrases that may help to manage stress more effectively:

I am mellow.
I don't fight; I flow.
I chill in the hot times.
Easy does it.

The Bible is a wonderful textbook for life management in general and for managing stress in particular. The Bible teaches that we should focus our thoughts on things that are good, pure, respected, and healthy. Focus your mind on phrases that feel relaxing to you. If you keep on repeating them they will take effect in your life.

You can learn to relax.

Day 5: Breathe

Breathing is obviously essential to life. We all do it automatically, but we don't always do it well. You can get more efficient use of your breathing with a little conscious practice.

Begin each day with a few deep breaths and some kind of relaxation exercise. You might want to remain in that relaxed state for a period of meditation or devotions.

Meditation by one definition means "murmuring to yourself" about things that are important to you. You might meditate on your goals, your values, your faith or something else beautiful. Taking charge of your thoughts and consciously focusing on pleasant things is one step in stress management.

Close the day with a time of deep breathing and relaxation. The more you practice relaxing, the better you'll become at it. The more you develop this skill, the more control you will be able to exercise over stress.

I am a person who relaxes and meditates daily. I believe it and I act on that belief. I have more energy when I engage in regular relaxation. That is probably because stress requires energy, so when I am more free of stress I am more energized. You can be more energized, too.

You can learn to relax.

Day 6: Do What You Can

Your life will be less stressed when you refuse to put pressure on yourself. No one else can effectively pressure you into higher levels of tension if you refuse to permit it. You can talk yourself into or out of internal pressure.

I often remind myself that, "I can only do what I can do and that is all that I can do." This is such a simple fact that I often forget it. I just cannot do more than I can do. Another way of stating this is, "I will do today what I do today." Of course I set goals for myself and pursue them. I just remind myself that my goals are my goals and not my gods. Few of the goals in life are absolutes.

I am not suggesting apathy. Have you ever heard anyone say, "I used to be apathetic but now I just don't care"? That's not the idea I want you to come away with. The idea is to focus on what you can realistically do.

A friend said to me that the secret of success is to lower your goals to the level of your achievement. He was only slightly exaggerating. The gap between your goals and your achievement is often filled with frustration, discouragement, and stress. You can reduce that gap in two ways. You can either raise the level of your achievement or lower the level of your goals. There is nothing wrong with either path. Lowering the level of your goals will reduce your stress—and you can always raise them again.

One of the steps in managing stress is accepting the responsibility for managing your expectations. Expect to do well but do not expect perfection. Reduce your expectations and you will reduce your stress.

You can learn to relax.

Day 7: Ask the Right Questions

If you listen closely you will hear a lot of people telling you what you "should" be doing. "Shoulds" are sure-fire stress producers. An effective way to manage the stress produced by "shoulds" is to ask questions. A wonderful question for the next person who tells you what you "should" do is, "Who says?"

Then others come and say, "Well, you certainly could be doing a lot better." Well, maybe. But better isn't always best! The right question for responding to this statement might be "So what?" One friend likes that question so much that he and his wife had a personalized license plate made with "SO WHAT" printed on it. Another bought a bracelet for his wife with the words, "So What?" engraved on it.

The way my father and others have asked this question is, "What difference will this make a hundred years from now?" I am certain that most of the things we become upset about are really not worth dying for. We take ourselves far too seriously. Life is very important but not all that serious.

So mellow out. Today commit yourself to doing what you can do today. It's all you will do.

I can only do what I can do.

I am only one person, but I am one.

So what?

Who says?

You can control and manage your stress by saying the right things to yourself and by asking good questions. The quality of the answers you get in life will have more to do with the quality of your questions than anything else.

You can learn to relax.

Week 5

Thoughts for Step Five: Develop Good Nutrition

Day 1: God and Food

We are just beginning to discover some of the wisdom in the Old Testament laws about food. Leviticus contains detailed religious laws about eating, and it relates obedience of dietary laws to faithfulness to God.

Leviticus 3:14-17 gives a specific instruction about fat. This passage simply says that people were to eat no animal fat or blood at any time or any place. Leviticus 7:22-15 instructs the Israelites never to eat the fat of cattle, sheep or goats. Pork was considered totally unacceptable, probably in part because of its high fat content.

We now know that there was dietary wisdom in those laws. In fact, most dieticians seem to agree that the number one nutritional problem in America is animal fat. Recommendations for your caloric intake from fat range down from 30 percent. Personally, I aim at an intake of less than 20 percent fat. The suggestion I see most often is that we should eat no more than 50 grams of animal fat per day.

While you would be wise to read books on nutrition, you'd be even wiser if you read the labels on the foods you eat. Even if you eat "fast foods" you can find the fat content in what you eat and keep it to a minimum. Fat comes to us in butter, margarine, sour cream, deep fried food, grease, hamburgers, cheese, and a host of other foods. Know your fats and avoid them.

Think about this: What you eat is even more important than how much you eat. Eat less fat.

Eating habits are vital to health.

Day 2: Eating Right

"A little sleep, a little slumber, a little folding of the hands to rest, and poverty will come on you like a bandit, and scarcity like an armed man" (Proverbs 24:33-34). The wise writer of Proverbs is explaining the wisdom of remaining vigilant, alert.

This is especially good advice when it comes to eating. "Just a day or two of eating junk, just a little yielding to the grease and fat, then your cholesterol will come as a robber and your clogged arteries like an armed man" (Bill Little 57:10). Okay, so that's my version! But the point is, don't become apathetic about your eating habits.

Short-term diets are seldom the answer for better health. Permanent changes in eating style are at least partial answers. Cutting back on fat content in eating, even for a little while, is better than not cutting back at all, but the best results come from permanent cutbacks on animal fat.

Here are some guidelines for eating that I have found helpful:

1. Eat wholesome, fresh foods, low in fat, high in complex carbohydrates and fiber, with not too much protein and with very low levels of salt.
2. Eat healthy snacks between meals. Snacks do not have to be junk food. They can be apples, oranges, bananas, bran muffins and even fat-free sweets on occasion.

3. Consciously and consistently control the fat in your diet (as we've just talked about).
4. Consciously and consistently control the cholesterol in your diet. Think of cholesterol in the same way you think of cigarette smoking. It does little good and clogs your system.
5. Learn to eat more slowly and chew your food better.
6. Learn to drink more water.

List in your journal the things you want to achieve in your own eating style.

Eating habits are vital to health.

Day 3: Enough Is Not Too Much

Everything in moderation is key in eating for health and disease prevention. Overeating is a serious health problem. There is no question that many people dig their graves with their teeth. In fact, the writer of Proverbs calls gluttony one of the seven deadly sins. He makes the extreme statement: "Put a knife to your throat if you are given to gluttony" (Proverbs 23:2). This is not a weight-loss recommendation. It is meant to emphasize control of appetite.

Not only is overeating a problem, but the kind of foods we eat present problems. You probably already know what to eat: high-fiber foods, low-fat foods, vegetables, grains, fruit. There is a whole new world of eating open to you, and it can be healthy.

Food is the fuel of life. It is important to eat the right foods and not just any foods. Good thoughts are food to the soul, but not just any thoughts. Think good thoughts and eat good, healthy food. You will be taking steps toward health and wholeness.

Eating habits are vital to health.

Day 4: Habits

The elimination of damaging habits is a vital step to take toward health and wholeness. And some of those habits are related to eating. One of these is drinking alcohol. While the Bible suggests moderation, it also calls attention to the problem of drinking, especially for pregnant women. The mother of Samson was instructed not to drink any wine during her pregnancy (Judges 13:14). This was long before we knew anything about Fetal Alcohol Syndrome (FAS). This is now known to be a leading cause of infant retardation.

When I think of damaging habits related to eating I also think of smoking. Many people connect smoking with eating. Some have pre-meal cigarettes and after-meal cigarettes. Some claim they cannot stop smoking because they would eat too much.

Probably no habit in American culture makes less sense and does more damage for the amount of benefit one receives than cigarette smoking. There can no longer be any debate by reasonable people concerning the devastating effects of smoking. Smoking not only damages the smoker, but we know now that people who breathe the smoker's smoke are also at greater risk than people who do not breathe it. We call this "passive smoking or secondhand smoke." Some of us are not being so passive about it any longer. I am not passive about breathing someone else's smoke. I ask for no-smoking seats and call attention to those who violate that space.

You must control your own habits. You developed them and you are responsible for controlling them. If a habit is hurting your health, why not write the name of that habit in your notebook? Can you stop such habits for your health's sake?

Eating habits are vital to health.

Day 5: The Easy Way Is the Hardest

In habits of eating as in so much of life, the easy way turns out to be the hardest, and the hard way the easiest. For example: When a student needs to study it may be easier at the moment to watch television, but on test day that decision turns out to be the hardest.

It may be easier to eat junk foods and even unhealthy snacks. It is certainly faster. The price? We develop tastes in ourselves and our children for less healthy foods. That may be too high a price to pay for convenience.

Old habits die hard, so you may want to start by changing just one meal a day for a few weeks. Take the time to prepare at least one meal that is high in fiber and low in fat each day for the next month. After that, you may decide to add one more. Or, instead of changing a second meal, change the snacks. Put out grapes, bananas, apples, some nuts, salt-free pretzels, and even bran muffins. It will help you to develop a habit with which you can live.

Is it difficult? Yes. The easy way usually leads to destruction (Matthew 7:13-14). The hard way is the easiest!

Eating habits are vital to health.

Day 6: Does Anyone Eat Right?

Does anyone actually follow all these eating guidelines? Yes, at least one group does. I'm not in accord with all of the theology of the Seventh-Day Adventists, but they do follow literally the laws from the Old Testament concerning diet.

The results are dramatic. As a group, Seventh-Day Adventists have half the rate of diabetes and uterine cancer as the general population. They have less than one half the rate of heart disease than the rest of this country has. These results are enough of a clue for me. I care about my own health enough to pay the price of watching my diet. It isn't really that difficult. Once you form the habit of reading labels and honestly commit yourself to seeking a healthier lifestyle, you can do it.

When you pray for good health you would be wise to add to the prayer a list of the things you are presently doing about your own diet. You can have good health if you cooperate with the good health guidelines available to you.

I hope that you will take the time to sit down and write out a list of the things you are doing to improve your own health. Be sure to include on that list some of the ways you are improving eating habits.

Eating habits are vital to health.

Day 7: Another Thought on Moderation

Philippians 4:5 says, "Let your moderation be known to all" (KJV). You don't have to become a fanatic about foods or anything else. Balance is usually healthy.

Americans seem to have a great deal of difficulty with moderation. We seem to be all-or-nothing thinkers and doers. My grandfather was given some medication by his physician. He was given instructions as to how he should take the medicine. Grandpa took the whole bottle the first day. He had a terrible reaction.

When his physician asked why he took it all at one time, Grandpa said, "Well, I figured that if a little bit would do a little good then a whole lot would do a lot of good."

That kind of "reasoning" seems to be alive and well today, even though Grandpa isn't. You don't have to eliminate all fat. You can eat up to 50 grams a day. You may eat as much as 2,000 or more milligrams of salt per day unless instructed otherwise by your physician. You probably need to eat about 30 grams of fiber every day.

Use good judgment. Read labels. Read reputable books on nutrition and diet. Talk to knowledgeable physicians about nutrition. Become conscious of your need for a balanced diet and do something about it.

Eating habits are vital to health.

Week 6

Thoughts for Step Six: Celebrate Life

Day 1: Fun and Energy

Years ago I read a book titled *How Never to Be Tired*. The premise of the book was that when you have fun you have lots of energy. You feel better.

My own experience supports this concept. My health is better, my energy is higher, and my enthusiasm is greater when I am having fun. I really have fun with my life. So true is this that many people around me think I only do what I enjoy. The fact is that I sincerely attempt to enjoy what I have to do.

I suppose it would be appropriate to call this the "psychology of joy" or the "theology of joy." The Bible is filled with the concept of joy. Philippians 4:4 says, "Rejoice in the Lord always. I will say it again: Rejoice!" Even in the face of problems and persecution the Christian is admonished to be happy and rejoice. Matthew 5:12 says, "Rejoice and be glad, because great is your reward in heaven." And then there is this statement in James 1:2: "Consider it pure joy . . . whenever you face trials of many kinds."

No matter what happens you can find a way to rejoice because of your faith. You can also have a lot of fun along the way. All you have to do is take it one day at a time.

Learn to smile. They say it increases your face value. Smiling is honestly contagious. Someone once said, "Smile and the world smiles with you. Cry and you just get wet." Fun is contagiously healthy. Get infected with laughter and joy.

Who doesn't love to spend time with fun people? You're the one who chooses your company, so choose to be with people who smile a lot and are able to see the humor in their circumstances. One way to insure having a healthier life is to invest in humor.

Having fun is healthy.

Day 2: Practice Rejoicing

Scripture admonishes us to rejoice without ceasing (Philippians 4). But rejoicing takes practice. Having fun requires commitment and practice. There are so many people around us who want to steal our joy that we have to practice not letting them do it.

Some people do a lot of complaining about their work, their families, their lot in life, their race, their gender, their country. These people are carriers of an emotional, if not physical, disease. Their sickness is contagious; sooner or later they steal joy from others.

It is not just in complaining that people attempt to steal others' joy. Some goad others into arguments, engendering angry and defensive feelings. I'm committed not to let the joy-stealers take away my rejoicing in life. I do not want to give them that kind of negative power over my emotions and my health.

I am committed to having fun and rejoicing. One of the things that helps me with this is asking myself the right questions. I have learned to stop asking myself, "How can I do this?" I now ask, "How can I have fun doing this?"

Most of the time you can find a way to have fun. Not everyone realizes this. I heard a woman say to her child at church, "Stop laughing, we're in church." She squelched her child's enthusiasm. Church is the most appropriate place for joy!

Sure, life is sometimes a real hassle. Don't let that stop you. Barbara Johnson said, "Don't lose your head in the battle, because you won't have any place to put your helmet."

Having fun is healthy.

Day 3: Laughable Quotables

I like to collect sayings and ideas that bring a smile to my face—or a good laugh. It's especially cheering to read a good quantity of them at once. I begin to laugh, and when I get going the laughter comes more and more quickly. I love to share the fun, so here is some of the "wisdom" I find humorous.

From Allen Klein:

> A California judge ruled that a man on trial for being an accessory to murder could go free because he was actually the murderer and thus could not be his own accessory. . . .
>
> A city in Michigan spent $50,000 on new flagpoles and then ran out of money, so could not afford flags for them. . . .
>
> A "Buy Britain" essay contest in England gave out radios made in Japan as prizes. . . .

From children:

> Three kinds of blood vessels are arteries, veins, and caterpillars. . . .

In many states murderers are put to death by electrolysis. . . .

From parents:

My son is under doctor's care and should not take fiscal ed. Please execute him. . . .

Please excuse Ralph from school on Friday. He had very loose vowels. . . .

Anonymous letter to county department:

I am very much annoyed to find you have branded my son illiterate. This is a dirty lie, as I was married a week before he was born.

From popular Christian author Barbara Johnson:

These days it takes nerves of steel just to be neurotic. . . .

I don't know where this one came from but I like it:

It rains on the just and the unjust but it rains more on the just because the unjust steals the just's umbrella.

When it comes to finding joy in life, a lot of people are apathetic. I care about health and I care about having fun.
Having fun is healthy.

Day 4: Laughter Eases Pain

We are great procrastinators. We frequently wait until a deadline forces us into action. We may never think about getting rid of pain until we have a severe pain, but that is far too late. The time to learn about pain control is before the pain develops.

One great pain controller is laughter. There are at least four ways that laughter helps us control pain.

1. Laughter distracts our attention. It takes our minds off pain and even creates some anesthesia. The pain is dimmed for us because so much of our attention is elsewhere.
2. Laughter reduces our tension. Muscular pain is intensified by tension. Laughing causes our muscles to relax, and relaxing them relieves pain.
3. Laughter changes our attitudes. Laughter serves as a kind of shock absorber that eases the bumps we get in life. I have had clients experiment with laughter to see how much it changed their moods. The effect is dramatic. It is hard to be depressed or anxious while laughing.
4. Laughter actually increases the body's production of its natural painkillers, endorphins. Some research indicates that laughter also causes the heart rate to increase and offers some of the same physical benefits of aerobic exercise. So, you see, laughing eases pain and substitutes to some degree for other forms of exercise. And it's free! What a way to reduce health-care costs!

Having fun is healthy.

Day 5: Fun Is a Spiritual Value

It is your mindset and not your circumstances that determines the level of joy that you experience in life. An especially dramatic, true illustration of joy despite circumstances is found in the biblical book of Philippians. Philippians is a letter written by the Apostle Paul just after an episode in his life of agonizing pain. Paul had been stoned and left for dead. He had been beaten for refusing to stop teaching about Christ. When he wrote the letter to the Philippians, Paul was in a Roman prison.

Yet the letter to the Philippians resounds with the theme of joy and laughter. Paul's sense of joy was deep because of his understanding of God. In chapter one, verses 3-4, Paul says he offers prayer "with joy." In the second chapter, verses 1-2, he asks the Philippians to be united in their thoughts and commitments to God in order to "make my [Paul's] joy complete." He urges the Philippians to "be glad" and receive his friend Epaphroditus "with great joy" (Philippians 2:28-29). In this little book Paul urges the readers to "rejoice in the Lord." He says that he has "rejoice[d] greatly in the Lord " (4:4, 10).

When I think of Paul's personal joy, I am amazed and encouraged. If a man facing prison could continue to rejoice, then I can rejoice in my circumstances. Part of spiritual maturity is being able to rejoice, to laugh no matter what our outward circumstances. "Rejoice in the Lord always. Again I say, 'rejoice,'" teaches Paul.

Having fun is healthy.

Day 6: Laughter Makes You Feel Better

Laverne came to me recently to discuss her feelings of anxiety and some physical pain she was having in her stomach. She was taking medication, but nothing was helping.

I had already given her a relaxation tape with some soothing music on it, which she was using on a regular basis. Laverne was also exercising for about thirty minutes every day. Her major problem seemed to be obsessive negative thinking that led to internal stress. She frowned constantly.

I encouraged Laverne to stop at a video rental store and pick out some of the funniest tapes she could find. She chose some Bill Cosby tapes. I urged her to watch the tapes at home for about an hour, really let herself laugh, and then call me to tell me how she was feeling.

She did not call until the next day. She had watched the tapes, and her stomach pain had subsided. She slept better than she had for some time. When she called she was clearly convinced that laughing had helped her feel better.

Laughing at something really funny takes your mind and your focus off yourself. It may be that self-centeredness is the major block to humor. Certainly it is a block to laughing at yourself. It takes a bit of selflessness to do that. Once you learn to laugh at yourself, you'll always have a funny person with you. You can help yourself feel better anytime.

Having fun is healthy.

Day 7: Five Reasons Humor Is Important

I want to make five points about the value of humor. These may be repetitious, but it's always helpful to review.

1. *Laughter is healthy.* This has been documented by Norman Cousins and others. The result is that "Laugh Centers" have sprung up all across this country. You can become healthier by learning to laugh more. Pay attention to the things that make you laugh.
2. *Laughter is a tension reducer.* Dr. William Fry of Stanford University calls laughter "a form of internal jogging." Laughter stimulates the cardiovascular system and actually exercises the lungs.
3. *Laughter is a pain reliever.* It distracts your attention away from pain. It reduces much of the stress and tension that add to your pain. It even stimulates

the production of endorphins, natural pain killers, in your body.
4. *Certainly, humor (laughter) relieves stress.* When you are able to laugh and joke about a life situation, you separate yourself from that situation and reduce its power to produce stress.
5. *You will have more friends if you learn to laugh.* People like to be around people with a good sense of humor.

It make take some practice, but you can learn to laugh! Having fun is healthy.

Week 7

Thoughts for Step Seven: Envision Wholeness

Day 1: Envision Health

Images are widely accepted as having tremendous impact on our lives. What we become is often believed to be the consequence of what we have imagined, dreamed, or envisioned. However, only in the last decade has adequate attention been given to the power of imagery in health, and efforts have been made to teach people how to use images to enhance the body's ability to heal. The Simontons popularized the concept in their work with cancer patients and their subsequent book, *Getting Well Again*.

For the last fifteen years I have used the notion of imaging to assist professional athletes in sharpening their skills. It is now a popular approach. I have also used this idea in helping people relax and in helping salespersons increase their confidence and productivity. More and more people are using imagery to influence their health.

Proverbs 29:18 says, "Where there is no vision the people perish" (KJV). If you see no future and nothing for yourself in the future, it will be hard for you to believe in tomorrow. How can you believe what you cannot imagine?

I believe I can become a healthier person by envisioning myself as a healthy person. I like to picture myself feeling good, walking, jogging, playing basketball, and having fun. What I picture tends to become reality.

This is not something evil or, as some say, "of the devil." This is a skill that puts God-given abilities to work. Maybe empowered, divine imagination was what enabled Jesus to see a withered arm become whole and then to make it whole. Our imagination is not divine, but is God-given.

If you're a nervous, anxious person, you might simply picture yourself calmly smiling and doing the things that usually bring stress. Close your eyes, take a few deep breaths, and see in your mind's eye your stomach becoming smooth and relaxed, inside and out. It just takes practice. Write down what image you are going to practice, and then start using your God-given imagination!

You may become what you see.

Day 2: Getting the Picture

This use of mental pictures is given various names: visualizing, imaging, seeing with the mind's eye, VMBR (Visual Motor Behavior Rehearsal), and convert modeling. There are other names, but the process and its acceptance are the same. The basic steps in visualization are these:

1. Select a goal, either a skill that you wish to develop or perhaps a healthier body or a well-functioning immune system.
2. Do deep breathing and progressive relaxation of your mind and body. You might use tapes to guide you through this process of relaxation.
3. Vividly envision your goal. Be as specific and clear as possible. Imagine clearly and distinctly.
4. Finish by affirming this image in your mind. You might draw pictures of yourself or your goals—or of yourself achieving your goals.

Using imagination is an area that comes naturally for children. Scripture teaches that we are to become as little children or we will never enter the kingdom of God (Matthew 18:3). Children are not afraid to use their imaginations.

If you cannot believe a thing in your head, how can you believe it in your heart? Imagine yourself strong and healthy. Perhaps you will become what you imagine. Get the picture?

You become what you see.

Day 3: Must You See What You Envision?

For a long time I was frustrated because while I was teaching others to visualize, I had a terrible time doing it myself. At least that's what I thought. In one seminar I complained to the leader, "When I close my eyes, I only see darkness. I can't see pictures of anything."

Jack said, "Sure you can. You just don't know that you can." He then instructed me to close my eyes and imagine myself in a living room with a new couch. He suggested that I pretend to lie down on the couch and relax. I did what he suggested and said, "I still don't see anything."

"What color is the couch?" Jack casually asked the question.

I didn't even hesitate. "Black."

"How do you know it's black?"

"I see . . ." I paused, and the group laughed with understanding. I saw more than I realized.

A cancer patient recently told me he was not coming in for any more training. He said, "This visualizing doesn't work for me. I can't do it. I see nothing when I close my eyes."

I had failed to make it clear to him that even when he did not *see* clear pictures he could still use his imagination. If this has been a problem for you, try the exercise Jack tried on me. Do you imagine that you can do that?

You become what you see.

Day 4: A Great Secret

Earl Nightingale wrote of his "greatest discovery." He said it was summed up in six words: "We become what we think about." Nightingale included visualizing in the thinking process. As he put it, "Visualization is a force of incalculable power. . . . We grow into our expectations. It's too bad that so few manage to muster expectations that are in keeping with their true potential" (Earl Nightingale, *Greatest Discovery*, p. 8).

For profit, salespeople are taught to use their thoughts and imaginations. Should you do less for your health? If salespeople can achieve success by holding an image of their goals in mind, couldn't you achieve health by holding images of health in your mind? I believe you can.

Why are we so afraid to use our imaginations? Perhaps it is because we have lost our ability to be like children. Jesus said that the kingdom of heaven belongs to those who are like children (Matthew 19:14). Perhaps one of the reasons that children can see the kingdom of heaven is that they can still use their imaginations. We lose a huge segment of life when we throw away our imaginations.

Others may refuse to use imagination because they associate it with evil. It is not the imagination that is evil, but what we do with it. In Genesis 6:5 we are told that people were condemned, not because they had imaginations ("inclinations of the thoughts of [their] hearts"), but because their imaginations were on evil continually ("only evil all the time"). Why not imagine, or picture, a world of love, beauty and health? We can't even imagine the great things that are in store for us (1 Corinthians 2:9).

In my Bible concordance the word *mind* is followed by the words *imagination* and *thought* as synonyms. Perhaps it would be easier for us if we read Philippians 2:5 "Let this mind [imagination] be in you, which was also in Christ Jesus" (KJV). The loss and misuse of imagination can lead to sickness. Someone once said, "Worry is the misuse of imagination."

Philip Bailey said, "We live in . . . thoughts, not breaths. He most lives who thinks most." I would add, "They best live, who think best."

You become what you see.

Day 5: Most Valuable Skill

What is the most important skill you can develop and teach to others? I know that teaching people to manage their thoughts and develop positive belief systems is vital, but I would probably say the skill most important to learn is that of managing images. I doubt any of us truly realizes how important it is to keep control of mental pictures.

If you become the things you imagine, wouldn't you be wise to develop greater control over that process? In a chapter entitled "Making Champions of Your Children," Stephen Covey writes of the value of mental images. He says that one of the skills that assist our children in becoming champions is the skill of imagining. "We teach them to visualize to help them realize their own potential" *(Principle Centered Leadership,* p. 148).

When I was very young, perhaps thirteen years old, I started envisioning my goals. I even drew pictures of myself reaching my goals. I credit that practice with much of the fulfillment that I have enjoyed in my life.

Use imagination. It is a valuable skill. It is an art to be regained.

You become what you see.

Day 6: It Is an Old Idea

The idea that you become what you envision is an old one, but it is as fresh as today's rain. Paracelsus was a Renaissance physician who is considered the father of modern drug therapy and scientific medicine. Nevertheless, Paracelsus opposed separating the spiritual from the healing process. He is quoted from the 1500s as saying, "Man has a visible and an invisible workshop. The visible one is his body, the invisible one is imagination [mind]. . . . The imagination is sun in the soul of man. . . . It calls the forms of the soul into existence." He also wrote, "The power of the imagination is a great factor in medicine. It may produce diseases in man . . . and it may cure them. . . . Ills of the body may be cured by physical remedies or by the power of the spirit acting through the soul."

We say it differently today, but the ideas about imagination are the same. What we see in our minds will have a dramatic impact on our bodies and our behavior. The apostle Paul said that we are to worship with our bodies and be transformed by the renewing of our minds (Romans 12:1-2). To be transformed means to be changed, but changed how? By the renewing of our minds!

Using the imagination is a skill that requires practice. I relax, concentrate on a specific goal, then imagine myself reaching that goal. I pray for God's help in achieving it. I see myself as I will look when I achieve it. I sense how I will feel when I reach it. I use my God-given imagination.

You become what you see.

Day 7: A Modern-Day Paracelsus

Coloring outside the lines is scary to us. When people follow a path that's unfamiliar or not accepted by others, we tend to be afraid of them. Jesus Christ was not willing to stay inside the lines. He taught almost everything in parables.

Thoughts for Step Seven

Glenn Clark said of Christ that he could look at a withered arm and see it as whole. He could look at people and see them as they could be as his redeemed followers. He had a parabolic way of viewing life. Christ used his ability to see the world as it could be.

Periodically someone comes along and tries to get us to open our minds to some old truths with new twists. Carl Simonton is one of those people. I think of him as a modern-day Paracelsus.

Simonton's technique begins with teaching a cancer patient to relax. The patient is then instructed to envision a peaceful, natural scene. Then the patient is told to see his cancer in his mind's eye and to picture his immune system working the way it's supposed to work. Patients are instructed to imagine an army of white blood cells coming in, swarming over the cancer, and carrying off the malignant cells that have been killed by radiation or chemotherapy. Just before the end of the exercise, the patient is to picture himself or herself well.

It is clear from the work of the Simontons that a person's mental pictures can play a fundamental role in disease. Do you want to be well and stay well? Then use every positive technique you can to achieve this goal. Imagine yourself well. Get the picture?

You become what you see.

Week 8

Thoughts for Step Eight: Exercise Healthy Spirituality

Day 1: Believe

Believe in something or someone greater than yourself. Every system of recovery I know of calls on people to have a faith in something. Members of Alcoholics Anonymous are admonished to trust in their "Higher Power."

Believing in Someone greater than ourselves is our source of hope and courage. Hope and courage are characteristics of healthy lifestyles. There are many times of suffering when believing in something more is all that keeps one going. The edge that makes the difference for many people who make it through difficult times is personal faith. Just as faith helps you make it through when you are sick, it can also help you stay healthy.

Faith is not just an emergency action. You've probably heard the old saying, "There are no atheists in foxholes." I'd add, "There are few in Intensive Care Units either." Don't wait for an emergency; begin to deepen your faith right now.

"Now faith is being sure of what we hope for and certain of what we do not see" (Hebrews 11:1). Hope and faith are constant companions, and hope is one of the healthiest and most encouraging of all emotions.

Faith in God is healthy.

Day 2: Faith and Forgiveness

Can there be any doubt that there is a relationship between a sense of forgiveness and a condition of wellness? Most of us recognize the devastating power of guilt. We don't need Freud to tell us about it.

Jesus Christ recognized the connection between forgiveness and joy. He said to a paralyzed man who needed healing, "Take heart, son; your sins are forgiven" (Matthew 9:2). Jesus then healed him.

Guilt produces stress. Stress retards our immune systems, and that can make us sick. One of the variables in preventing disease is a sense of being forgiven. This is one area where faith can have a tremendously powerful influence on our health. Our faith in Christ is the source of forgiveness. We need to seek the forgiveness of God and then make a concentrated effort to forgive ourselves.

One of the most honest bumper stickers that I have seen is the one that says, "Christians are not perfect, just forgiven." I am forgiven. So are you if you believe. Remind yourself each day: "I am forgiven, and I forgive myself." Healthy faith leads to forgiveness, and forgiveness leads to better health.

Healthy faith is healthy.

Day 3: Being Forgiven Means Being Forgiving

Glenn Clark observed that "it is the most spiritually sensitive, the very finest souls amongst us, who suffer reaction from wrong thinking much more quickly than the thicker-skinned brand of humanity."

Selfishness, thoughts of self or focus on self, may be the grandfather of the diseases related to sensitivity. Anger and fear are the parents. If this is true then we need to move away from selfishness, anger, and fear to have a better chance at preventing disease.

Selfishness hangs on to hurt feelings. It harbors resentment and refuses to forgive. An unforgiving attitude is a terrible block in the flow of life. It can become an obsession. Healthy spirituality leads us not only to be forgiven, but also to forgive others.

I can illustrate one of the negative impacts of unforgiveness from my own life. For many years I held a grudge against the president of my college for cancelling my basketball scholarship because I was a married student and it cost more to give a married student a scholarship than to give one to a single student.

I harbored resentment toward him for at least twenty years. I never talked about it to anyone, but I would sometimes dream about that situation. There were times it would come to my mind in the middle of the night. That resentment cost me rest and sleep. It never affected the college president at all.

About ten years ago, I had occasion to share these feelings with a group of friends. I confessed my feelings to them and made a commitment to let go of my resentment. I consciously made a statement of forgiveness to that man. It was a religious commitment for me.

I have not lost any more sleep, and I no longer feel the resentment. I am learning that forgiving others is as important as being forgiven myself. That has been good for my health.

Healthy faith is healthy.

Day 4: Faith, a Sign of Strength

We are often tempted to believe that faith is a sign of weakness. Some even go so far as to call it "an opiate of the people." But, in fact, faith is so fundamental to life that it must be a part of every healing system in the world.

Everyone believes in something or someone. I make no apology for my faith. There was a time when I did. I wanted to appear intelligent. I thought this would be hindered if I admitted that I believed in God.

In retrospect I see that I would have been a greater influence for healing if I'd had more courage in expressing my personal faith in God. I gradually began to get the picture. Society made it perfectly acceptable to express faith in gurus, soothsayers, astrologists, psychics, channelers, or any weirdo who came up with a philosophy, but not so acceptable to express orthodox faith in God.

Far from a sign of weakness or ignorance, though, healthy faith is an expression of strength and intelligence. Some of the strongest personalities in history have been people of deep religious faith: Abraham, Moses, Abraham Lincoln, Martin Luther, Martin Luther King, Jr., and the list goes on. The point here is that faith is a resource for our health. We must not be afraid to express it.

Healthy faith is healthy.

Day 5: Real Power for Health

There is one central idea that every religion has taught and every would-be savior has exemplified. "It is, that belief determines your experience. What you are on the inside determines what you experience on the outside. Your faith in good increases your area of good. Your faith in negatives, which is fear, increases your problems" (Barker in *The Science of Successful Living,* p. 1).

"Your faith has healed you. Go in peace and be freed from your suffering," said Jesus (Mark 5:34). Leslie Brandt says even Christians who believe in a Christ of love and come to him with confessions and prayers for forgiveness and healing "are still assailed by guilt-feelings, plagued with weaknesses, defeated and overcome with failures, incapacitated by tragedies, and very much in doubt about the outcome of it all. The reason? Perhaps our touch has not really been the touch of faith. We may be jostling Christ rather than embracing Him" *(Meditations Now,* p. 206).

Health is greatly improved by meditating on the positive characteristics of God. Even if you don't yet believe in God, you may be helped by permitting yourself to meditate on the divine characteristics. They include, love, acceptance, forgiveness, peace, joy, hope, courage, righteousness, justice, and many others. Read your Bible for more, especially the Psalms.

One friend of mine used to meditate on one of those words each day. He would start the week by making "love" his word for the day. That day he looked for every expression of love he could find. The next day he looked for acceptance, etc. It was an exercise in healthy thinking.

Healthy faith is healthy.

Day 6: Faith and Courage

There are times when living absolutely calls for courage. When you have a difficult situation to face, your first temptation is to run away and hide somewhere. Say you made a mistake at work and have to face a supervisor. Or someone is angry at you and you have to confront the situation. Or maybe you are called to the hospital to the bedside of a loved one. There are hundreds of situations like these in a lifetime.

When you are afraid, your body is stressed. The immune system doesn't function properly and you become sick. The fact is that there are times of fear for all of us. There are times when we are called on simply to put one foot in front of the other and just keep on going. Those are the times that can crush our souls. Those are the times when we need the courage that comes from personal faith.

The apostle Paul said, "We are always confident.... We live by faith, not by sight" (2 Corinthians 5:6-7). We can face the difficulties with courage because we believe in God. The same faith that is required to help me meet the major disasters and trials is required to help me meet the daily challenges. Courage for daily living is based on personal faith.

I believe in God; therefore I will not fear any confrontation in this world. I will walk by faith.

Healthy faith is healthy.

Day 7: Thoughts about Spiritual Things

Glenn Clark said that Jesus had the ability to see the world as it was and then dream or imagine it the way it could be. He could look at a withered hand and imagine it whole, and it would be whole. He could say to the paralyzed man, "Arise, take up your pallet, and walk" (John 5:8, NASB). Can we look at what is and with our imaginations try to see what could be?

Sit down in a quiet place. Take a deep breath and relax. Now imagine a world that is filled with peace and love—like the world described in Isaiah 11:6-8 where the calf and the lion and the lamb lie down together. See in your mind Black people and White people walking hand in hand and smiling as they walk. See a homeless person being invited into the home of someone who is wealthy. See yourself doing an act of kindness for someone in need, and remember the words of Matthew 25:40, "Whatever you did for one of the least of these brothers of mine, you did for me."

Think of your own body as whole. Imagine yourself walking and leaping and celebrating life. See your back straight and feel the clean air fill your lungs as you breathe deeply.

After spending some time doing this, ask yourself, "Are these things I have been imagining or thinking, lovely, pure, good, and healthy?" If so then, "think about such things" (Philippians 4:8).

There is something powerful in expressing, imagining, or thinking about honest personal faith in God. I will never be reluctant to express my faith. It is good for my health. It is God for my health.

Healthy faith is healthy.

Appendix B

Special Guide for Cancer Patients

The sense of helplessness that many cancer patients feel is the most debilitating effect of our society's attitude toward the disease. Many people who must face the diagnosis feel that they can only lie back and suffer whatever cancer dishes out. Some even refuse medical treatment, believing that passive acceptance or active refusal are their only options.

This is not true. You can fight cancer by becoming an active participant in your treatment program. What follows is a summary of the principles taught at The Cancer Support Center to all patients who enter the program. By applying the principles described in this guide, patients become working partners with the rest of their medical team to fight the disease in their bodies. As you will see, these principles are the same ones that have been described in this book.

These principles sound so commonplace that they may not appear to be therapeutic. They are so worn with use that you might overlook them as you search for support and comfort. It is their very usefulness that has made them seem commonplace, for they are part of every wise person's life.

People are healthier if they practice regular relaxation. Relaxation helps people who are sick to "go with the flow" and to put their energy into recovery.

Focusing on health and envisioning healing helps people prevent and fight off disease. Our dreams have a way of coming true. Dreams of wholeness give us power for healing.

Active participation in our own health care allows us to cease feeling victimized and to begin working toward health.

A clear faith in a Power greater than ourselves benefits our health. A clear life philosophy deepens our experience and helps us to stay well.

Laughter and fun are not trivial distractions. They are as much a part of life's whole as are tears and sorrow. You'll live longer and be healthier if you enjoy life.

Positive attitudes and thoughts empower us to attain health.

A high-fiber, low-fat, regulated diet is healthy. If we eat right, we live longer and healthier.

Love and encouragement buoy us up. We were made to love one another. We need to help others along the way and to seek out people who do the same for us.

Hope and a sense of purpose pull us onward. If we have something to live for, we may live longer, and our lives will certainly be more worth living. Hope ties everything else together.

Special Guide for Cancer Patients

No one questions the seriousness of the disease of cancer. We who work with cancer patients know that your body will need all the energy you can summon to fight this invader. If you learn how to reduce tension, fear, depression, and other energy-draining emotions, however, your body will marshall its forces more effectively and focus them on fighting the cancer.

The purpose of the program described in this booklet is to help you reduce the need to deal with stress and negative emotions, to help you recover vitality and hope, and to assist you in learning techniques that will enable you to cooperate with whatever treatment you are receiving. We believe that this will help you to make the best possible use of your body's natural resources.

We also want to help you improve the quality of your life. It isn't only that we want you to live more fully whatever time you have left, even though that is a worthy goal for all of us. We also believe that, as the quality of your life improves, your enjoyment of life will increase, your desire to live will intensify, and you will use up less energy coping with despair and anxiety. The result will be not only a fuller life, but a longer life, and, in some cases, the restoration of health.

How much this program will help you is largely up to you. It will not be enough merely to read the guide. You must make the commitment to practice what you learn with all the dedication of the most devoted religionists in the world or with the discipline of a serious athlete. It is not enough to know. You must also do!

The principles recommended here can work to make your life better and longer. The major question may be whether you want improved health enough to really work at this program, one day at a time. If you do, then you can expect positive results in your life. We are asking you to approach these instructions with devotion and determination.

This plan is "An Adjunct Treatment Program for Cancer Patients." It is called "adjunct" because it supplements whatever regular or conventional treatment, such as radiation or chemotherapy, you are receiving. This program is not a substitute for other treatments. All of your doctors, nurses, technicians, psychologists, clergy, and others are working with you as a team, fighting the cancer that has invaded your body.

This program is called "treatment," but it might just as accurately be called "education" or "training." We want to help you aid your medical treatment through education and training.

There are four strands in this program: relaxation, visualization, new ways of thinking, and exercise. You will be on your own in applying what you learn. We cannot motivate you to do what you are unwilling to do, but remember that we are asking you to work as if your life depended on what you do. In fact, it may.

1. Relaxation training. The first element of the program is a technique that, with practice, will help you relax. We begin here because this tool will enable you to control stress and tension. All of us experience tension to some degree and can profit from learning to release it, but the purpose here is more than easing present tensions. We want to help you learn a technique, a tool, that you can call upon whenever you experience tension of any kind. A relaxed body is freer to function normally. Relaxation also reduces pain. And people are more open to learning other new techniques when they are relaxed.

The relaxation technique described here is an effective one, well-tested in the laboratory and clinical practice. It involves sitting in a quiet place and practicing the relaxation of your muscles in groups, beginning with your facial muscles and going through the other muscles all the way to your feet.

It is common knowledge that stress reduces the body's resistance to disease. Research suggests that excessive stress increases certain hormones that retard the immune system. It stands to reason that, if stress reduces resistance, it also impedes recovery from disease. If you learn to relax, your body will be free to fight the cancer.

One woman in our pilot study found that relaxation relieved the nausea she had experienced before, during, and after her chemotherapy treatments. In her case, nausea was caused more by tension resulting from fear than by the chemotherapy drugs. Other positive effects will undoubtedly result from the use of relaxation techniques.

Relaxation is something you can achieve. It is something you can do on your own, as well, a place where you can begin to participate in your own health. Make an audio tape of the following instructions, or ask someone to read them slowly for you as you respond, step by step. Use the tape at least twice a day until you have learned the instructions. The relaxation process should last about ten to twelve minutes.

> Find a quiet, comfortable place.
> Sit or lie down and close your eyes.
> Take a deep breath and hold it for about five seconds, then slowly release it.
> Breathe normally for a moment and say to yourself, "When I inhale, I breathe in relaxation. When I exhale, I breathe out tension."
> Breathe in relaxation and health, breathe out tension and impurities.
> Now take another deep breath. Hold it for about five seconds and slowly release it.
> Let you body relax. Think of it as a bag filled with sand.
> Let your muscles fall apart.
> Take your time, and become conscious of the muscles in your forehead. Briefly raise your eyebrows up toward the top of your head, and let them fall.
> Let the relaxation begin to flow down your face.

Think of the muscles around your eyes. Squint briefly, then let your eyes relax.

Move your attention to the muscles in your jaws. Clench your jaws briefly, then let them relax.

Focus your attention on your neck. Move your head from side to side, then let it tilt forward if you are sitting, or fall back if you are lying down.

Think of your shoulders. Shrug them up toward your ears and let them fall.

Feel the relaxation that started in your forehead flow down over your face and into your neck and through your shoulders into your upper arms.

Tighten the muscles in your upper arms briefly, then let them relax.

Think of your lower arms. Make fists, then let your fingers straighten until the relaxation seems to drain through them.

Roll your shoulders forward to stretch the muscles in your back. Let the muscles relax.

Think of your chest. Push it out briefly, then let it relax.

Push your stomach toward your back, then let it out.

Imagine that your stomach is like a pile of soft rubber bands.

Arch your lower back forward, then let it relax.

Tighten your hip muscles, then let them relax.

Think of the muscles in your upper legs. Tighten them briefly, then let them relax.

Think of your lower legs. Lift your toes toward your knees, and then push them down. Now relax.

Let every muscle in your body just fall apart as you take a deep breath and slowly release it.

Now you can open your eyes at your own pace and go about doing whatever you want to do.

If you wish, you are ready now to practice mental imaging.

When you have mastered this exercise, you probably will be able to induce a relaxed state by simply closing your eyes and taking a deep breath or by imagining a relaxing scene. Use this skill when you are receiving treatments. It can also help you sleep more restfully.

2. *Positive imaging.* The process of envisioning a goal is not new. Scientists have used it to solve problems. Baseball players have improved their pitching accuracy and raised their batting averages by imagining themselves succeeding. The idea of fighting cancer with this method, however, is relatively new.

Imagination and mental pictures can accomplish truly amazing results. People who see themselves running activate the muscles in their legs; laboratory instruments have measured these contractions. In other experiments, human beings have altered body processes such as brain wave patterns and blood pressure, by means of mental imagery. Young men in another study dramatically improved their performance in darts and basketball free-throws, solely by means of mental practice.

These skills are applicable in any area of life. You can use them to fight cancer. The idea is to imagine your own body and your medical treatment effectively fighting, controlling, and even destroying the cancer in your body. Create a mental picture of your white blood corpuscles attacking and killing cancer cells, your radiation therapy effectively hitting its targets, and your chemotherapy doing its job efficiently. See your own body's defense system consciously cooperating with your treatments to destroy cancer in your body.

The evidence indicates that positive imagery helps. Even if it did nothing else, it would at least help you believe that the destruction of cancer cells is possible. To "see" it is to be able to believe it! This belief increases your hope. Hope displaces despair and thus helps you relax and use your energy for healing. Every time you practice your relaxation exercise, use your imagination to see the very thing you actually want to happen. This discipline could be compared to a game of "let's pretend," but it is not a game, and it is not just pretending. It is envisioning a potential reality.

Not only will this help raise your hope, it will deepen your relaxation and make it easier for your whole system to cooperate in fighting cancer. Remember, once again, that the technique will benefit you only if you do it, at least twice a day.

3. Changing your thinking. "Cognitive restructuring" is a fancy name for changing the way you think. You can employ a variety of thinking techniques to help you deal with fears, frustrations, pain, depression, and expectations. This is another thing you can do yourself, a skill you can apply in any area of your life.

Basically you are learning to rethink your fundamental beliefs about yourself and the world. At one point in your life, you learned to think and believe as you do. Your reactions are not automatic by nature; they are learned. As children, we hear something, repeat it in our thoughts, and silently file it away for future reference. We learn through repetition. Using the same process by which you learned your ideas in the first place, you can substitute more realistic, helpful, and positive ways to think and react.

Some of the things we learned as children are false and may, in fact, harm us. We may have learned to believe crippling things about ourselves. We often become unwitting fulfillers of our own negative prophecies.

As an example of how our thinking affects the course of our lives, imagine two people who have lost their jobs. The first person reacts to the experience by becoming depressed and suicidal. The second may be disappointed, but nevertheless vigorously pursues a new job. The experience affects them differently because they believe different things about the situation and talk to themselves in different ways.

"Oh, my gosh, I've lost my job," the first person says. "I'm a failure. I'll never get another job. My life is not worth living." Such thinking naturally leads to depression.

The second person sees things differently. "Well, I lost my job. That's bad, but it is not the end. I can work, and I'll start looking tomorrow." This sort of thinking leads not to depression, but to a new job!

Something happens to you. You talk to yourself about it, and discuss your beliefs with yourself. Then you react according to your internal discussion. The same kind of process occurs when your doctor tells you that you have cancer. You begin to go over your beliefs. You may say, "Oh no! I've got cancer. There is no hope for me. I'm going to die right away, and I probably will have a lot of pain and disfigurement." If you believe and say that, the result is despair, depression, and panic.

You may honestly believe these statements, but they are not necessarily true. Suppose you say something different to yourself: "I have cancer. That's bad, but it isn't the end of the world. As long as I can fight, there is hope. I will do everything I can to overcome this thing. Life is fickle anyway, and anyone may die at any time. My problem is to make my life as full and meaningful and healthy as possible. Now let me see. What can I do now to help myself?"

If you react to your bad news with such beliefs, you are likely to feel a lot better. The point is that if you learn to change your beliefs and the way you discuss them with yourself, you can change the way you feel. Emotions can be controlled.

We are not proposing that you put on a happy face and pretend to be stoic and brave. In fact, expressing the emotions you really do feel is important to your recovery. We are not urging you to embrace positive ideas that are untrue, just because they're positive. That kind of pretense won't do you any good. But you can change the prophecies of doom and other beliefs you have that are negative and false, because they damage you.

The process is simple. First, become aware of your present beliefs about yourself, the world, and other people. Pull into your mind the thoughts that make you frightened, tense, and depressed. Part of becoming conscious of your emotions is being completely honest and open about them. Are you angry? Do you hold some resentment? Do you feel guilty? Are you afraid? Are there other feelings you have never dealt with honestly? Face these things.

When you identify an emotion that has to do with cancer, take a private inventory to find out what beliefs generated that emotion. What are you saying internally? Whatever it is, write down that belief. It is a hypothesis about your situation. Now that you have it identified, examine it. Do a little research. Check with your physicians to see whether your information is correct. If not, then write down the new information.

Begin to make two lists. Write any negative original belief you may have about yourself and your disease on the left side of a page. Across from each old belief, on the right side of the page, revise the belief; state the original idea in a more positive way.

Now learn the list on the right side of the page. Say these statements aloud. Memorize the new beliefs. Use them as often as you can. Say them to your friends and relatives. Whenever you think the old thought, replace it with the new one. Use the old only as a stimulus for the new. You are now consciously changing your thoughts. As you do so, the emotions, fears, frustrations, depressions, and general misery associated with the old ideas will change too. Teach yourself new ideas. They will change your emotions.

Any kind of emotion can be dealt with in this way, for feelings are usually the result of our beliefs. Examine the thoughts behind it, write down the thoughts or beliefs, check them to see if they are really valid, then rewrite them in more positive words.

The lists that follow will help you get started, if you want to change your fears of cancer or death, your depression, your sense of helplessness.

If you suffer from depression, keep a list for a week of all the depressing thoughts you notice. You may hear yourself saying these things aloud, or you may be aware of the fact that you are saying them to yourself. Write the depressing thoughts on the left side of the page. Then, on the right side of the page, opposite each negative thought, write a more positive or encouraging way to interpret the same topic, and write that statement on the right side of the page. Examples are listed below.

Depressive Thought	**Positive Thought**
No one cares what happens to me.	Some people care what happens to me. I care!
Nothing good ever happens to me.	Some good things happen to me, and a lot more good can happen.
I'm sick and I'm going to die.	Everyone is going to die and none of us knows when. But I can live whatever life I have as fully as possible.
People make me miserable.	I have been making myself miserable, and I can stop it.

If you have trouble thinking of positive statements, ask a trusted friend to help you verbalize the positive or encouraging statements.

An additional skill will help you deal with other difficult emotions. Learn to formulate statements that you can say to yourself. Fear, for example, is a universal human experience. It cannot be denied away, but it can be confronted. First, become aware of your fears and the experiences that produce them. When you have identified your fear, use the following guide for help in confronting and coping with it. These are statements you might repeat to yourself. You may want to add other statements of your own. Some of the statements that follow will help you when you anticipate something that makes you fearful, others when you are experiencing a present fear.

When you feel fear or know you are facing a fear-producing event:

"I'll describe my fear or what I have to do."
"I can think of a plan to deal with it."
"I'll think about what I can do. That's better than getting anxious."
"I'm not going to make negative statements to myself."
"I'll think through this rationally."
"I won't worry. Worry doesn't help."
"I will face this thing and I'll make it!"

When the fear is present or a "fear event" is taking place:

"I'll 'psych' myself up. I can meet this challenge."
"I'll reason it away."
"One step at a time I can handle this situation."
"I won't concentrate on fear. I'll think of what I can do."
"I'll relax. I'm in control. I'll take a deep breath."
"I'll label my fear from 0 to 10 and watch it change."
"I won't try to eliminate fear totally; just keep it manageable."
"I'll pause now and focus on the present."

After you have coped with your fear, reinforce yourself:

"It worked; I did it!"
"My ideas—they are the problem. When I control them I do all right."
"Wait until I tell my friends about this!"

Pain is another universal human experience. All of us have felt pain in the past and will certainly experience more. You can help yourself deal with pain by preparing yourself for it. Practice the following statements, or devise statements of your own and practice them.

Preparing for pain:

"What is it that I have to do?"
"I can develop a plan to deal with this."
"I'll think about what I can do."
"I won't worry. Worry doesn't help."
"There are a lot of strategies I can call upon."

Confronting and handling pain:

"I can meet this challenge."
"One step at a time, I can handle this situation."
"I'll stop thinking of pain and think instead about what I can do."
"I'll relax, take a deep breath, and use one of my strategies."
"I'll relax. I'm in control. Now I'll breathe deeply."
"This pain just reminds me to use my new skills."

Coping with feelings at critical moments:

"When the pain comes, I'll pause and keep focusing on what I can do."

"I am thinking, 'What is it I have to do?'"
"I won't try to eliminate pain totally, just keep it under control."
"If pain mounts, I can switch strategies and stay in control."

When you feel relief from pain:

"Good, I did it."
"I handled that pretty well."
"I knew I could do it."
"Wait until I tell my friends about this."

Pain may generate stress. If you have pain, you need a strategy for coping with it. Select one of the following coping strategies, and use it as part of your plan.

Attention diversion: Focus your attention on things other than your pain. Do mental arithmetic, for example. Study the pattern in your clothing. Count ceiling tiles. Find any activity that requires your concentration and focus on that activity.

Somatization: Focus your attention on your bodily processesor sensations. For example, observe and analyze the feelings in your body that may result from the pain you are experiencing.

Image manipulations: Change or transform the experience of pain by means of imagery. Use your imagination to create a fantasy story that is incompatible with pain. Imagine that you are doing something you enjoy, like lying on a beach in the sun. Or imaginatively transform your pain into a fantasy that includes pain but minimizes the sensation. For example, imagine that you are feeling cold or numbness, rather than pain. Or use your imagination to transform the context of your pain. Take an experience that includes pain, and change the context. Imagine, for example, that you are feeling a pulled muscle as you cross the goal line for a touchdown, or a gunshot wound you have received while in the line of duty for your country.

If none of these strategies feels comfortable or natural, develop your own method.

4. Exercise. The fourth strand in this training program is more than a fad in America. It is an essential element in any person's health program. Proper exercise keeps our blood circulating freely and helps us breathe easier. It seems that our bodies are made for exercise. Research has indicated for seventy years that active bodies more effectively resist and fight cancer. Tissues from fatigued muscles in mice have been shown to retard cancer.

We are not suggesting that you overdo exercise, of course. Use your own good judgment to tailor the following guidelines into an exercise routine that fits your own needs.

- Set aside one hour at least three times per week.
- If you have not been exercising, use light exercise like walking and simple movement of your arms.
- Increase your exercise gradually and use as a guideline your ability to converse while doing it. As long as you can maintain a conversation, you are probably within safe limits.
- Choose your own exercises, but make them light enough to continue for the full hour.
- Carry on normal activities as much as you can.

When people are sick, they are usually told to rest, but too much rest can, in some cases, be detrimental. Remember that you are responsible for your own program. You can do it. Only you can do it.

Both relaxation and exercise relieve stress. Here are several additional ideas that may also be helpful, and you may come up with others.

Learn to ask the right questions. When you meet a situation that has produced anger, frustration, or depression in the past, take a deep breath and ask yourself, "How do I want to respond to this situation?"

Learn to put things in perspective with important questions like: "Who says?" "So what?" Or the big one, "Is this worth dying for?" You never get good answers until you ask the right questions.

Have fun! Consciously choose to have as much fun as you possibly can. If you can make a situation laughable, do it. Laughter can heal.

Keep variety in your life. Try new things, eat new foods, go to new places, try new hobbies, or just change your daily schedule. Variety reduces stress. If you carry a suitcase in one hand, that arm and hand become stressed. Change hands!

Practice your religious faith. If your faith is positive, it will relieve stress. Take the responsibility for finding and expressing your own faith or philosophy. It is your right.

Exercise, relax, have fun, spice your life with variety, and find your own meaningful faith. Whatever their circumstances, people who do these things find that their lives improve. That is true for young people, old people, people in good health, and people with cancer.

You need not abandon your life and accept whatever happens, like a sacrificial lamb. You can take charge of yourself, in ways this guide suggests. If you do that, you will undergo the trials of medical treatment with higher spirits than you ever thought you could muster. As an active member of the team, you will make the most of the treatment plan. And you will come through it with a new pride in your own personal power.

All good wishes to you on your journey!

Printed in the United States
43372LVS00005B/1-102